# CONTROLLING DIABETES THE EASY WAY

STANLEY MIRSKY, M.D.,

AND

JOAN RATTNER HEILMAN

# CONTROLLING DIABETES THE EASY WAY

*THIRD EDITION*

RANDOM HOUSE

NEW YORK

This book cannot and must not replace hands-on medical care or the specific advice of your doctor. Use it instead to help you ask the right questions, make the right choices, and work more closely with your doctor and other members of your health-care team.

All rights reserved under International and Pan-American Copyright
Conventions. Published in the United States by
Random House, Inc., New York, and simultaneously in Canada
by Random House of Canada Limited, Toronto.
Earlier editions of this work were published in 1981 and 1985
by Random House, Inc.

LIBRARY OF CONGRESS CATALOGING-IN-PUBLICATION DATA
Mirsky, Stanley
Controlling diabetes the easy way / Stanley Mirsky and Joan
Rattner Heilman.
p.      cm.
Includes index.
ISBN 0-679-77803-9 (pbk.)
1. Diabetes—Popular works. I. Heilman, Joan Rattner.
II. Title.
RC660.4.M55   1998        616.4′62—dc21        97-23426

Random House website address: www.randomhouse.com

Printed in the United States of America on acid-free paper
98765

*To Susan, Jennifer, and Jonathan*

*Also to the memory of my mentor,*
*Dr. Elliott P. Joslin, 1869–1962.*

*Gladly would he learn, and gladly teach.*

# CONTENTS

|  | Introduction | ix |
|---|---|---|
| 1 | What It Means to Be a Diabetic | 3 |
| 2 | Are You a Hypoglycemic? | 17 |
| 3 | Making the Diagnosis for Diabetes | 23 |
| 4 | Nobody Loves a Diet | 31 |
| 5 | Exercise: Essential for Diabetics | 83 |
| 6 | Taking Oral Agents | 95 |
| 7 | Going the Insulin Route | 107 |
| 8 | Testing Your Blood Sugar | 130 |
| 9 | Insulin Reactions | 142 |
| 10 | Coping with Acidosis | 153 |
| 11 | Worries, Worries, Worries: The Chances of Diabetic Complications | 158 |
| 12 | Rules for Sick Days | 188 |
| 13 | Watching Your Feet | 197 |
| 14 | Pregnancy Problems | 205 |
| 15 | Sex and the Diabetic | 220 |
| 16 | Traveling: Diabetics on the Move | 227 |

17  Can Diabetes Be Prevented?          239
    Resources                           243
    Other Useful Resources              244
    Index                               245

# INTRODUCTION

Even though diabetes is one of the most common chronic diseases, it has never been easy for the millions of diabetics to find rational answers to their questions about it. For many people, their condition seems to present a situation so complicated that they are overwhelmed and confused. They feel dominated by the diagnosis and the lifestyle it often imposes.

The purpose of this book is to counter the misconceptions and fears about diabetes, to give straightforward, easy-to-understand explanations of what this age-old disease actually is, where it comes from, how to cope with it, and how to minimize its effect on your life.

It's impossible to know too much about your diabetes. The more you know, the more control you will have over your own destiny. For this is a disease that requires you to be your own doctor much of the time.

In this book you will find clear information about every aspect of diabetes, with special emphasis on diet—your major weapon. I have been a specialist in diabetes for many years, and recommend for what to many is the simplest, easiest, most effective diet plan ever proposed for controlling blood sugar. It is so easy, in fact, that you have only to remember just one rule and know how to count to fifty.

Included also is a special chapter for hypoglycemics—people who suffer from low blood sugar. Though hypoglycemics are not diabetics, they, too, have a problem maintaining a normal blood-sugar level, and will therefore also benefit from the same diet plan.

— Stanley Mirsky, M.D.,
New York, 1998

# CONTROLLING DIABETES THE EASY WAY

# 1

# WHAT IT MEANS TO
# BE A DIABETIC

Nobody is delighted to be diagnosed as a diabetic. After all, diabetes is a chronic disease with serious consequences and complications if it isn't kept under control. You must watch what you eat, get regular exercise, and maybe take pills or insulin injections. It is a condition that you will have for the rest of your days. So far, there is no cure.

But diabetes is the one major disorder whose effects on your lifestyle depend to a remarkable degree on how much you know, and how much effort and time you are willing to spend paying attention to it. You can minimize the impact it has on your daily life as well as your future health simply by learning all about it and then living with a few rules that actually would make everyone in the world healthier if they, too, abided by them. At best, you may lose all evidence of diabetes and indeed the disease itself. At least, you may be able to reduce the amount of medication you require—all as the result of eating sensibly. The easy-to-follow plan presented here may change your life.

About 16 million Americans are diabetic (though half of them don't know it), and 1,800 new cases are diagnosed every day. Diabetes and its complications are responsible for more than 400,000 deaths a year, making it the fourth leading cause of death by disease.

Studies estimate the cost of diabetes to be about $92 billion a year—$45 billion in direct costs, including hospitalization and treatment, and the rest in lost productivity, disability payments, loss of work time, and premature deaths.

To give you all the bad news at once, diabetics are much more likely than others to become blind, lose a foot or a leg, have kidney failure, develop coronary heart disease, and have other difficulties.

Now for the good news. Tremendous progress has been made in only the last few years in the prevention and treatment of the disease. It is very likely that a cure will be discovered soon. Most diabetics who not long ago would have died at an early age or would have existed with such dire complications that life would have been hardly worth living, can now lead almost normal lives and can look forward to a respectable, reasonably healthy old age.

Here are some of the statistical facts about diabetes:

• More than nine out of ten of the 8 million diagnosed diabetics in the United States have type 2, or noninsulin-dependent diabetes mellitus (NIDDM). If they follow the correct diet, this group—formerly known as "adult-onset diabetics" because the disease usually strikes adults over the age of forty and most commonly over fifty-five—may never need insulin injections except perhaps during periods of stress. The remaining less than 10 percent of diagnosed diabetics have type 1, or insulin-dependent diabetes mellitus (IDDM). Once called "juvenile-onset diabetics," this latter group will always require insulin and cannot get along with diet alone or even with oral antidiabetic agents. Type 1 and type 2 are two separate disorders, although they share many of the very same problems.

• All type 1 diabetics require insulin injections.

• Ten to 20 percent of the diagnosed type 2 diabetics are treated with diet and exercise. Thirty to 40 percent take oral drugs to keep their blood sugar within acceptable limits. And

30 to 40 percent require insulin injections or a combination of insulin and oral medications.

• Type 1 diabetes is more prevalent among whites than other racial groups.

• About 6 percent of white Americans, age forty-five to seventy-four, have type 2 diabetes, according to the National Institutes of Health. Over 14 percent of older Hispanic Americans and 10 percent of African Americans have diabetes. African Americans, however, are twice as likely as whites to get type 2. And black women are particularly vulnerable: One in four over the age of fifty-five has diabetes.

Few Inuits and Asians living in their homelands have diabetes. However, the numbers rise markedly, especially for the Japanese, among those who make their homes in Hawaii and mainland United States.

Native Americans have the highest rates of diabetes in the world, about seven times higher than Caucasians.

• Women are twice as likely to get diabetes as men.

• The chances of developing diabetes double with every 20 percent of excess weight and with every 10 years of increasing age.

## WHAT IS DIABETES?

Diabetes mellitus is a metabolic disorder that results in persistent *hyper*glycemia—an abnormally high amount of sugar in the blood. (On the other hand, *hypoglycemia* means the opposite—an abnormally *low* blood-sugar level.) It is thought today that diabetes is actually several different diseases with different causes, all with the same result: the inability of the body to efficiently utilize the carbohydrates we eat as a source of fuel.

Glucose, the end product of carbohydrate metabolism, is the body's primary fuel. It is used immediately for energy, or it is stored in the liver in the form of glycogen to be called upon at a later time. When the body is unable to metabolize carbohydrates, which are derived mainly from sugars and starches, the blood becomes overloaded with glucose. The kidneys are unable to handle the excess and in most cases it "spills" into the urine.

## WHAT'S GONE WRONG?

If you have diabetes, something has gone awry in the elaborate system of metabolic checks and balances the normal body uses to maintain a safe blood-sugar level. Sometimes the pancreas, a large gland located on the left side under the ribs, completely abdicates its job of turning out insulin, the hormone that helps the cells to use glucose as their fuel. Sometimes the pancreas secretes an inadequate amount of insulin, not enough to cope with the carbohydrates you eat. And sometimes the pancreas is unable to "recognize" the high blood-sugar level and so does not produce enough insulin in response to it even though the capacity is there.

In most cases, however, especially in older overweight diabetics, the pancreas continues to produce plenty of insulin, often much more than normal. But the insulin cannot perform its function of helping the cells to use glucose. The reason is a shortage of insulin receptors, areas on the cell membranes that allow insulin to permeate the cell walls. A whole cell, for example, usually has about 30,000 receptors, of which about 10 percent, or 3,000, are at work at any one time. Research has found that, in a susceptible person, overeating and a large weight gain increase the production of insulin, which then causes a reduction in the number of receptors. Plentiful insulin floats uselessly in the blood, unable to penetrate the cells, while sugar piles up but cannot be utilized.

## HOW DOES YOUR BODY MAKE INSULIN?

Insulin is manufactured by complicated little biochemical "factories" in the pancreas. These are the beta cells, responsible for so much of our well-being. They are located in the islets of Langerhans, one to two million tiny areas of the pancreas comprising maybe 2 percent of the entire gland.

The islets also secrete other hormones—glucagon from the alpha cells, somatostatin from the delta cells, and amylin from the beta cells, for example—which are deposited along with insulin into the bloodstream via the tiny blood vessels that surround them. All of these hormones are involved in maintaining normal blood-sugar levels.

When it is working normally, the pancreas responds to every minute fluctuation in blood sugar, releasing insulin whenever it is needed just as a thermostat turns a furnace off and on to maintain a constant temperature in your house. When the blood sugar rises after we eat, a signal goes to the pancreas, alerting it to move some insulin out.

When there is not enough glucose in the bloodstream to be used for fuel, the liver, stimulated by the glucagon from the islets' alpha cells, releases glucose from its warehouse of stored glycogen. At the same time, amylin alters the sensitivity and secretion of insulin and may help slow the absorption of sugar through the intestines. When a sufficient amount of glucose has been secreted by the liver, somatostatin is responsible for turning off the production before it goes too high.

It takes most people about two to three hours to return to the normal fasting blood-sugar level after a high-carbohydrate meal.


## HOW IS INSULIN USED?

In the normal person, starches, sugars, and proteins (58 percent of which is eventually converted into carbohydrate), are broken down by the intestines into glucose, a form of sugar. The glucose is carried throughout the body by the bloodstream, entering the cells with the help of insulin, then burned for energy by the muscles. Some of the leftovers are stored in the muscle cells or converted into fat. The rest is stockpiled in the liver in the form of glycogen, to be called upon later if the blood sugar falls too low.

If there is not enough insulin or if the insulin available cannot help the glucose permeate the cells, this sugar accumulates in the blood, often in very high concentrations. The result is diabetes.

In a nondiabetic, glucose concentration is usually below 115 milligrams per 100 milliliters of blood plasma, and even after a huge overload of sugar rarely goes above 160 to 180 mgs. In uncontrolled diabetics, it can go much higher, frequently reaching 800 or even 1,000 mgs. Though there's obviously plenty of glucose available to feed the body's hungry tissues, it cannot be used effectively and the cells can literally starve, no matter how much you eat.

At the same time, the liver is stimulated to release its stores of sugar and then to begin a process called gluconeogenesis. In a response to an emergency call for more fuel, this important organ takes the huge amounts of amino acids produced by the starving tissues and changes them into more glucose. Fats are also transported to the liver. Now ketones, the end products of the burning of fat instead of carbohydrate for fuel, also overload the kidneys and spill into the urine. When this happens, and nothing is done to remedy the situation, the body lapses into a diabetic coma—a real emergency.

## TYPE 2 (NONINSULIN–DEPENDENT DIABETES MELLITUS, OR NIDDM)

About 92 percent of diabetics are NIDDM, or type 2. If you are in this category, you continue to manufacture insulin, perhaps not enough to cover your needs, or perhaps more than enough, but it cannot be efficiently utilized. You can probably control your diabetes with diet and exercise, or diet combined with oral hypoglycemic drugs that stimulate the release of insulin, delay the absorption of carbohydrates, or lower your blood sugar by suppressing the liver's output of glucose. Or you may require insulin injections to supplement your own supply.

Although your diabetes may have been discovered after you developed specific symptoms such as excessive thirst and urination, more likely you were diagnosed during a routine medical checkup. Or maybe your eye doctor or dentist was the first to suspect it. Most cases of type 2 occur gradually, and never present obvious warning signals.

Even teenagers may have this variety of diabetes (about 5 percent of type 2s are under twenty), but statistically it is probably likely to occur in people over forty, becoming more common by age fifty or sixty.

Most type 2s have inherited a tendency toward diabetes. Eighty-five percent have a diabetic parent or other close relative. Although the responsible genes have not yet been isolated, researchers have identified a protein called PC-1 that seems to shut down the insulin receptors, thereby decreasing insulin sensitivity.

What's more, they are almost always overweight. The vast majority of adult diabetics are too heavy or even obese. Many overweight type 2s can lose their diabetes by losing weight. Sometimes a loss of even a few pounds is sufficient to accomplish this miracle because now you may produce enough of your own insulin to keep your blood sugar normal or increase the number of cell receptor sites so that the insulin you produce can be utilized properly.

The number of receptors and the ability of the insulin to bind to them are also increased by exercise. In controlled studies, it has been discovered that regular, vigorous exercise can lower or even eliminate the need for pills or injections.

Not all type 2 diabetes, however, is the result of overweight in a predisposed person. Sometimes it's simply the result of an inefficient pancreas. The beta cells become unable to sense the sugar molecules and so can't respond accurately to their presence; or they simply cannot produce enough insulin. In these cases, losing weight won't help but eating correctly and exercising enough will, perhaps supplemented by oral agents or insulin.

## TYPE 1 (INSULIN-DEPENDENT DIABETES MELLITUS, OR IDDM)

Type 1 diabetes, once known as juvenile diabetes, is quite another story and may even be another disease with similar outcome. There are comparatively few IDDMs—less than 10 percent of the total number of diabetics.

Type 1 can strike at any age and about 15 to 20 percent of IDDMs are adults when they are diagnosed. But it happens for most people before they are twenty, and most commonly around the ages of eight, twelve, and puberty, when dramatic growth spurts take place. For every 100,000 people in the country, there are 50 diagnosed diabetics under the age of five; there are 150 under age ten; 270 below age fifteen; and 325 per 100,000 population by the age of eighteen.

If you are a type 1, you have a marked insufficiency in the number of beta cells your pancreas possesses and you produce little or no insulin of your own. That means you must take insulin injections to compensate. Except in extremely rare cases, the oral drugs, designed to stimulate production in a pancreas that has the capability to make its own insulin, won't work for you.

Unlike type 2, type 1 diabetes generally shows up very abruptly and dramatically, with unmistakable symptoms— excessive urination and thirst, dramatic weight loss, weakness, irritability. If these symptoms go untreated, they rapidly progress into acidosis (see Chapter 10) and finally coma in only a few days or weeks.

As a type 1, a person with the severest form of diabetes, you probably do not have diabetic parents, though there is a genetic factor here too, as studies with identical twins have shown. Far from overweight, you are probably very thin and perhaps wan. There is no way for you to lose your symptoms by losing weight and eating sanely. But supplementary insulin, aided by good diet and plenty of exercise, will keep your blood sugar relatively normal.

## THE CAUSES OF DIABETES

Heredity plays a very important role for the type 2s. We know there must be a genetic predisposition, perhaps resulting in early aging of the pancreatic cells or the shut down of insulin receptors. When some kind of stress—overweight or pregnancy, for example—is added to the genetic tendency, diabetes is the result. The sumo wrestlers of Japan are programmed to gain tremendous amounts of weight. They are adored by the sportsmen of Japan, but develop diabetes and heart disease early in their lives. They blaze like meteors across the sky, but the trip is short.

The genetically isolated Pima Indians who live in a remote river valley in the Arizona desert tend to be sedentary, overweight, and diabetic. Half of the Pimas over thirty-five have diabetes, 15 times the incidence among the general population in the United States, the highest rate ever recorded. Yet those Pimas who live in Mexico and work the land usually remain thin and do not have evidence of increased diabetes.

Both groups are good examples of the inherited tendencies toward this disease combined with obesity. If you have a family history of diabetes, it would be extremely wise not to get fat.

For the IDDM, the type 1 diabetic, the theory today is that the disease is triggered by a virus that infects the insulin-producing beta cells of a person whose genes make him or her vulnerable to developing diabetes. The infection then sets off an autoimmune reaction. This means that antibodies are produced in response to the infection, circulate in the bloodstream, react to pancreatic beta cells as if these cells were foreign invaders, and destroy them, knocking them permanently out of commission. The suspected triggering viruses include Coxsackie $B_4$, mumps, and German measles.

Many genetic markers for diabetes have been identified only recently. If a child has genes HLA-DR3 or HLA-DR4 on his sixth chromosome, inherited from *both* parents, he has 2½ times more chance of becoming a type 1 diabetic after a viral infection. Eighty-five to 90 percent of all type 1 diabetics have DR3 and/or DR4. And if aspartic acid is not found in position 57 in these genes, the risk of diabetes increases even more. But remember, even if a youngster has DR3 or DR4 genes, it is not inevitable that he or she will develop the disease.

Variants of another HLA gene may also play a role in this kind of diabetes. Researchers have recently found that DQA1 (0301) and DQB1 (0302), again on the sixth chromosome, are strong predictors of diabetes when passed along by two parents. Others—DQB1 (0201) and DQB1 (0301)—are protective against it.

A second indicator is the presence of cytoplasmic pancreatic-islet-cell antibodies, found in 80 to 90 percent of children destined to become diabetics. But if, like the Inuits, a child has B7 on the sixth chromosome, his chances of diabetes are decreased. And if he has DR2, it is extremely doubtful he will get diabetes. Though people with DR2 make up a quarter of the population, only a few cases of diabetes have ever been reported among them.

Occasionally, diabetes is the result of another physical condition: pancreatitis, tumors, adrenal imbalance, injury to or removal of the pancreas, or damage caused by several drugs.

## WHO GETS DIABETES?

Diabetes gives geneticists headaches because it is almost impossible to predict, even in the presence of defective genes, who will eventually become diabetic, although many risk factors have recently been determined (see Chapter 17).

It was once thought that all the children of two diabetic parents would eventually become diabetic. Today it is thought that 60 percent is a more accurate figure. With one diabetic parent, sibling, or child, there is a 3 percent chance of diabetes by the age of forty to fifty-nine, a 10 percent chance after sixty.

The identical twin of a person who becomes diabetic before forty has a 30 percent likelihood of developing the disease. If the disease has its onset after forty, the chance an identical twin will have it increases to close to 100 percent, but if the disease does not occur within three years, the identical twin's chances drop substantially. Fraternal twins, by the way, have about the same risk as other family members—about 10 percent.

## EVERYTHING'S UNDER CONTROL

Once you know you are diabetic, you've got a new goal in life: to keep your blood sugar as close to normal as you possibly can. That means, ideally, between 70 mgs percent fasting and 150 mgs after a meal. That's not easy, especially in times of stress when every diabetic's blood sugar runs rampant, but you can stay within that range most of the time if you remember your future depends on it.

For many years, it was thought that this "tight control" was not too important as long as you felt well and functioned normally. Today we know differently. Uncontrolled diabetes—consistently high blood sugars—can eventually affect every system of the body, resulting in many exotic varieties of diabetic complications. For example, people with diabetes are 2½ times more likely to suffer from strokes and 2 to 4 times more likely to develop cardiovascular disease. Over 60 percent of diabetics have high blood pressure and 60 to 70 percent have nerve disease. Diabetes is the leading cause of new cases of blindness in adults and of end-stage kidney disease. It is the primary cause of amputations, an estimated 54,000 of them a year in the U.S.

Those are frightening facts but here's the good news: Control your diabetes—in other words, maintain your blood sugar at consistently normal levels—and you can avoid or minimize all of these nasty complications. A thirty-year study of 4,400 diabetics revealed that those people who had held their blood-sugar levels to below 300 mgs had three times less risk of complications after fifteen years of the disease than those with higher levels. Those with a level below 250 mgs had 5 to 20 times less risk. And those who kept their blood sugar below 120 on diet alone had almost no risk of complications at all.

In 1998, the United Kingdom Prospective Diabetes Study strongly proved and confirmed an early DCCT study that intensive treatment—be it with oral agents (sulfonylureas or metformin) or insulin—reduced diabetic complications equally without one or the other more dangerous to the heart. The study also showed reducing blood pressure greatly reduced complications.

In a study of the Pimas, it was found that complications occurred in the group with fasting sugars above 140 and above 200 two hours after eating. The higher the sugar, the more likely the complications.

Of course, life is not fair. Some people who pay no attention to their control never develop complications in spite of their lack of vigilance, while others who exercise great care do get them in later years. But, in general, it is true that greater control means a better, healthier, longer life.

Nobody's perfect, and you won't be either. You will not always follow your diet plan, you will succumb to temptation now and then, you'll forget to test your blood sometimes, you will let your control get out of hand. But if this becomes your pattern and not just an occasional slip-up, you will undoubtedly pay the piper later. All the health problems associated with diabetes are hastened and exacerbated by poor control.

## WHO'S IN CHARGE AROUND HERE?

You are. Your doctor will diagnose and prescribe and direct your treatment, but you are the only one who can live your own life. You're the one who puts the food into your mouth, decides how much exercise to get, makes the blood tests every day, handles the crises of hypoglycemia and high blood sugar. You can get direction and advice from your doctor and this book, but you are in charge of yourself.

This does not mean you are out there all on your own. It is very important that you see your doctor frequently, whether or not you take insulin. The doctor monitors your blood-sugar control in order to prevent complications in the future, picks up early changes, works with you on problems concerning diet, exercise, lifestyle, or whatever, and advises you on handling illnesses.

If you are a diabetic who is regulated by diet alone, see your doctor *at least* every three months. Don't go whenever you feel like it, or only when trouble brews. Go regularly on a scheduled basis.

If you take oral agents or insulin, make an appointment even more often, depending on your condition. Once every one to three months is right for most people. Never skip or postpone an appointment if you can possibly avoid it. And don't hesitate to call your physician if you see a change in the results of your home glucose monitoring.

To find a doctor who can give you good care, call your local chapter of the American Diabetes Association or of the Juvenile Diabetes Foundation. You will be given the names of several doctors in your area who are the most knowledgeable about diabetes. This is a specialized field, and many general physicians are not qualified to handle your problems. Your future will be much brighter if you find a doctor who is.

Living with diabetes means a constant balancing act between the food you eat and the insulin you produce yourself or take by injection, along with the exercise you get. Insulin provides the mechanism for burning the food for energy to run your complex body. Exercise lowers your blood-sugar level. If you eat more food, you will need more insulin and exercise. If you eat less food, you will require less insulin and exercise. That's simple. What's hard is always having to think about this balancing act especially at times when, often through no fault of your own, this balance is thrown out of kilter.

For many people, one of the most trying aspects is the need to be consistent, to lead a structured life. Especially if you take insulin, you soon discover that you must eat a preordained amount of carbohydrate, that you must eat on time, take your medication on schedule, make constant blood tests, check in with your doctor regularly. While everyone else, it seems, can stay up all night partying, eating pizza, and drinking sodas, stuffing themselves one day and fasting the next, paying no attention to medicines or doctors, you, if you are on insulin, must plug along, day after day, on three meals plus two snacks.

That can be difficult, but it will pay off. Consistency isn't such a tremendous price to pay for feeling well now and in the future. It will eventually become a lifestyle you can live with.

# 2

# ARE YOU A HYPOGLYCEMIC?

The word *hypo*glycemia simply means "low blood sugar," nothing more or less. (Hyperglycemia—diabetes—is the opposite, meaning "high blood sugar.") The number of people diagnosed as hypoglycemics has grown to enormous proportions in the last few years. In reality a rare phenomenon (except as an insulin reaction among diabetics), hypoglycemia has been blamed for a variety of strange feelings and symptoms that seem to require a label and an explanation, has made fortunes for many doctors, nutritionists, and quacks, and has been both overdiagnosed and underdiagnosed. We all know people who have been told, or have decided, they have chronic low blood sugar. Most of them could not honestly be called hypoglycemic. On the other hand, there are unsuspecting people who do have consistent low blood sugar at times during the day, who suffer from symptoms as a result, are often called neurotic, and who have not been correctly diagnosed as actually having hypoglycemia, a condition, not a disease.

A "normal" blood sugar (fasting or over three hours after a meal) is considered to be between 70 and 110 mgs percent (7 to 11 parts glucose to one hundred parts of blood), a level that remains fairly constant because of the interaction of intestinal absorption, the liver, and the pancreas.

But many people have blood sugars that drop much lower, perhaps to 40 to 50 mgs percent, and cannot be called hypoglycemic. So, how low is too low? And when does a specific number spell out hypoglycemia?

These are not easy questions to answer, but in general, a blood sugar below 50 mgs percent *that coincides with other symptoms* means you are hypoglycemic. Some people have no symptoms when their sugar is low; others may have the symptoms of hypoglycemia when their blood sugar is quite normal. No diagnosis of hypoglycemia can be made unless low blood sugar and specific symptoms *occur simultaneously*.

## THE SYMPTOMS

Hypoglycemia is not dangerous, but it can make your life miserable. The symptoms may (and may not) include general weakness, fatigue, inability to concentrate, listlessness, butterfly sensations in the stomach, subnormal temperature. Also, rapid heart rate, shakiness and palpitations, sweating, and apprehension. As someone has described it, it's as if you have almost been hit by a train.

Some hypoglycemics experience headaches, irritability, double vision, nausea, tingling, drowsiness, slurred speech, and an irresistible urge to yawn. These are all associated with a low supply of glucose to the brain, which needs sugar to function. Very low drops in blood sugar can produce balance and hearing problems. Unsuccessful pregnancies have also been ascribed to hypoglycemia. In Australia, a study revealed a high incidence of perinatal deaths, as well as small placentas and small babies, among mothers who had low blood sugars. Hypoglycemia can be a powerful appetite stimulant. Many hypoglycemics gain large amounts of weight as a result.

True hypoglycemia can be compared to trying to run an eight-cylinder car on two cylinders and often is the reason for depression.

## THE TREATMENT

There is only one way at the present time to treat hypoglycemia, and that is with diet. Except in a very occasional case with an organic origin, no other treatments or medications are of any value, including injections, megavitamins, and hair analysis (which will only reveal what kind of shampoo you are using). In a few years, there may be other treatments—for example, Pramalintide, an analog of human amylin that is produced by the beta cells, and certain oral agents now used to treat diabetes. Pramalintide, now being tested, seems to help prevent blood sugar from going way up and then rebounding to very low sugar and all its symptoms. In addition, some of the oral antidiabetic agents—Glucophage, Precose, and perhaps others now in development—may well find a place in treating reactive hypoglycemics.

Usually wrongly proposed for this condition is a low-carbohydrate, multiple-meals-a-day diet with an inordinate amount of fats and proteins, and insufficient carbohydrate for body fuel. This diet is not only difficult for most people to follow but, over the years, it can load up the arteries with fatty plaque.

The diet that works best for hypoglycemics is the same diet we recommend for diabetics. Read Chapter 4 and you will see how easy it is to live with this sensible, rational food plan that simply limits quickly absorbed sugars and offers the same proportion of other carbohydrates typically eaten by Americans. With it, you will avoid the unsettling periods of reactive low blood sugar and its symptoms.

## AN EXPLANATION OF THIS PHENOMENON

Hypoglycemia is often the result of too much insulin produced by the pancreas in response to an overload of sugar into the bloodstream. It may be an overreaction of the body's blood-sugar regulating system. It tends to occur in families of diabetics, but that fact does not mean hypoglycemics will turn into diabetics one day. The current estimate is that about 50 percent of *true* hypoglycemics will one day be diabetic.

There are organic and nonorganic causes of the condition. The organic causes include tumors in the pancreas which then has no stop-and-go mechanism, allowing the beta cells to secrete insulin without regard for incoming sugar, and cirrhosis of the liver that results in little glycogen storage and glucose delivery when sugar levels fall as a result of not eating. Sometimes the adrenal glands are damaged and do not perform their vital function of converting protein into glucose for fuel. Removal of parts of the stomach may result in the "dumping syndrome." Without the normal sphincter tone at the lower end of the stomach, glucose is released too precipitously into the small intestine. So much glucose enters at once that insulin production cannot keep up and blood sugar rises. This triggers more insulin production, resulting in low blood sugar.

Alcoholism, too, can cause hypoglycemia. Alcohol interferes with the conversion of glucose from protein and inhibits the release of glucose from the liver's stores of glycogen. In fact, you needn't be an alcoholic but simply overindulge in order to have a hypoglycemic episode. A recent study involved ten patients who were given three double vodka martinis for lunch. Three of them developed not only the inability to concentrate, but hypoglycemic blood-sugar levels a few hours later.

But the usual variety of hypoglycemia is nonorganic and is an exaggerated response of the pancreas which, stimulated by large doses of sugar entering the bloodstream, pours out too much insulin. Usually, after a sugar overload, a reactive hypoglycemic experiences a rapid rise in blood sugar to higher-than-normal levels and then a quick drop to below normal two or three hours later. Sometimes, however, the blood sugar does not rise abnormally at first, but later falls below normal.

When the sugar drops very low, the symptoms may appear. If they do, you are hypoglycemic.

## DIAGNOSING HYPOGLYCEMIA

The best way to diagnose low blood sugar is with a glucose tolerance test, made in the doctor's office or a laboratory where results can be measured immediately after each of the several blood specimens are drawn.

The test involves drinking a large dose of glucose solution on an empty stomach and then having blood taken every hour up to five hours later. The blood is tested for glucose content. If you have hypoglycemic symptoms at any time between the scheduled testing hours, you must also be tested at that very moment. See Chapter 3 for more details.

Important: a glucose tolerance test will not give valid results if your pancreas is unprepared for it. For three or four days before the test, you *must* consume a normal amount of carbohydrate—at least 100 to 150 grams a day—so that your pancreas is not startled by the large load of sugar you will be given at one time. An unprepared pancreas can trigger a classic hypoglycemic reaction even among normal people.

Another way to test for hypoglycemia is to draw blood for testing at the moment you experience symptoms after eating a normal balanced meal. If your sugar is abnormally low at these times, then you are hypoglycemic.

## LIVING WITH HYPOGLYCEMIA

Let's make ourselves perfectly clear: there is now no treatment for hypoglycemia except *diet*. This does not mean you must avoid carbohydrates and eat mostly proteins and fats which may eventually clog your arteries. Instead, you should eat a balanced diet that consists of at least 50 to 60 percent carbohydrate. It is exactly the same food plan as a diabetic should follow.

Like diabetics, you should avoid sweets and too much quickly absorbed natural sugar that can overload the pancreas and stimulate it to pour out an excessive amount of insulin. You will probably do well on three meals a day, but if you feel better with snacks between meals there's no reason you can't have them.

The diet, described in detail in Chapter 4, will provide your body with the fuel it requires but won't overstimulate your pancreas and cause a hypoglycemic episode.

## HELPFUL HINTS

• It is wise to eat whenever you drink alcohol and to drink only moderately. Alcohol inhibits the release of glucose from the liver when it is needed by the body.

• If you are going to exercise strenuously, have a snack first. Exercise quickly depletes the blood sugar you have on board. If your vigorous activity extends over a long period of time, eat or drink some carbohydrate every hour or so.

• Coffee, tea, cocoa, chocolate, all in a chemical family called xanthines, seem to trigger hypoglycemic episodes for some people. The xanthines inhibit one of the enzymes whose function it is to tell the beta cells of the pancreas to stop producing excess insulin. So be sure to avoid these if this is true for you.

NOTE: In the remainder of this book, little else will be directed specifically to you, the hypoglycemic, though much of the information applies to you, especially in the chapters on exercise and diet. Eat properly, and your troubles will be over—it's as simple as that!

# 3

# MAKING THE
# DIAGNOSIS
# FOR DIABETES

To diagnose diabetes, your doctor must confirm through tests that you have inappropriately high blood sugar—sugar that rises to abnormal heights and stays there too long. In a nondiabetic, blood sugar rises and falls throughout the day, but never goes very high or very low because the pancreas secretes sufficient and efficient insulin.

## HOW IS DIABETES DISCOVERED?

Many people are diagnosed as diabetics when urine or blood tests are made during routine examinations. Their symptoms are so minor that they don't even notice them. In fact, they may have had diabetes for years without knowing it. Other diabetics are discovered by their dentists who find unexplained periodontal problems, their podiatrists who spot suspicious foot sores, ophthalmologists who notice vision changes, other doctors who are looking for the underlying reasons for recurring vaginal or urinary infections, male sexual problems, menstrual irregularity, early menopause, itching (especially in the genital or anal areas), tingling, numbness, or fatigue.

## THE OVERT SYMPTOMS

When diabetes occurs more suddenly or severely, the symptoms may be more sudden and severe too. These include the three "polys": polyuria, polydipsia, and polyphagia.

*Polyuria* is excessive urination (when it occurs at night, it is known as excessive nocturia), and a strong sense of urgency. When the carbohydrate you eat is not utilized, it is dumped into the urine to be excreted from the body. Urine is produced in vast amounts, the bladder fills quickly, and much of an uncontrolled diabetic's time is spent in the bathroom. In babies, an increased need for diaper changes may be an indication of a problem.

The huge loss of water from the body tissues causes dehydration. Diabetics develop *polydipsia,* a tremendous thirst that can never be satisfied.

*Polyphagia,* excessive hunger, is the least common of the three major symptoms. It represents the body's frantic attempt to get the fuel it requires. Even though large amounts of food may be consumed, there will be rapid weight loss. One patient, a marine sergeant, was diagnosed after he continued to lose weight even though he ate one or two pounds of meat and drank two quarts of milk and juice with every meal.

Other symptoms of diabetes include weakness, heaviness of the legs so that climbing stairs or hills becomes extremely difficult, subnormal temperature, slow healing, dizziness, acidosis, and, of course, diabetic coma.

Because uncontrolled diabetes is associated with an increased incidence of heart disease, blindness, miscarriage, and spontaneous abortion, these conditions may also raise in your doctor's mind the question of the possibility of diabetes.

## JUST A MATTER OF ROUTINE

Discovering hyperglycemia—high blood sugar—with a urine test during a routine physical examination is a matter of chance if you are not severely diabetic. The urine must be checked at just the right moment. Glucose is carried in the bloodstream and travels through the kidneys. Below a blood-sugar level of about 156 mgs percent, most people will not lose sugar in the urine and it will not be discovered during the test. Instead, it will be returned to the body through the renal veins, which transport blood from the kidneys back to the heart. If you have a large meal but not enough insulin, or if it is not used effectively, some sugar will turn up in the urine. But this won't happen until an hour or so after the meal, when the food has had time to be turned into glucose and has made its way to the bladder from the kidneys via the bloodstream.

Even with excess blood sugar, a test taken an hour after a meal may be so diluted with urine accumulated *before* the meal that the sugar won't show up in concentrated amounts. Two to three hours after the meal, however, the urine will reflect the higher blood sugars.

The speed of the blood flow to the kidneys also influences how much sugar appears in the urine. Sometimes, especially with diseases like heart failure, this rate drops, and, even though the sugar is high, even far above 156 mgs, very little escapes into the urine. The doctor making the diagnostic tests should take this high renal threshold into account.

In pregnancy, the reverse happens and there is an increased rate of blood flow to the kidneys. Now more sugar appears in the urine at *lower* levels. That means all pregnant women with sugar in the urine are not necessarily diabetic, though they should definitely be tested for the possibility.

## MAKING THE DIAGNOSIS FOR DIABETES

For many years the gold standard for the diagnosis of diabetes was the glucose tolerance test (GTT) which we will describe below, but it is gradually being replaced by a simpler, less expensive, and less time-consuming procedure, the fasting plasma glucose test.

## THE FASTING PLASMA GLUCOSE TEST

This test, now deemed sufficient for diagnosis by the American Diabetes Association, requires a sample of blood taken from your arm after you have had nothing but water for at least the previous eight hours. Your sugar level should be no higher than 126 mgs percent to be considered normal.

Sometimes another procedure is added: the two-hour postprandial plasma glucose test, when your blood sugar is measured two hours after a meal. If it is over 200 mgs percent, you will be classified as diabetic.

## HbA1c: THE GLYCOHEMOGLOBIN TEST

The purpose of a HbA1c test is to monitor blood-glucose control and it is not yet widely used for diagnosing diabetes, but you can be fairly sure you have diabetes if this test comes up with a higher-than-normal result. The HbA1c, a blood assay that requires only one blood sample taken at any time, no matter when you last ate, measures your level of glycated hemoglobin and reflects an average of your blood-sugar levels over the last two or three months.

Hemoglobin, a protein in red blood cells that carries oxygen to the body's cells, attaches to glucose in the bloodstream when glucose is elevated and stays attached for the life of the blood cell, about 120 days. It is this glycated hemoglobin that can be measured. If you have a glycated hemoglobin level of 7 percent or more (the norm in most laboratories is 3.2 to 6.2 percent), you can be classified as a diabetic, even without an official glucose tolerance test. When you get your report from the laboratory, remember that only the A1c value is relevant (some labs report other components as well).

The relationship of mean blood glucose (MBG) to A1c may be explained this way: MBG equals 30.9 glycohemoglobin (GHB) minus 60.6. In other words, every 1 percent change in GHB is associated with a blood glucose change of 31 mgs/dl.

At 7 percent the average blood glucose is 155.7 mgs/dl, and at 9 percent is 217.5 mgs/dl.

## THE GLUCOSE TOLERANCE TEST

Although the glucose tolerance test may soon become outmoded except for the diagnosis of hypoglycemia, it is still used by many doctors, clinics, and laboratories. Here's how it is done:

Before you have a glucose tolerance test, you *must* eat at least 100 to 150 grams of carbohydrate a day for at least *three* days. This is, for most people, a normal amount. If you have been eating very little carbohydrate, the glucose tolerance test will catch your pancreas unawares and the results may not be accurate.

Diuretics and estrogen supplements may also influence a glucose tolerance test interpretation. The test is best done in the morning, sitting down and relaxed. No smoking until it is completed.

On the morning of the test, you are asked to eat no breakfast. Your first blood sample will reflect a *fasting* state—no incoming food for at least the previous eight hours. The doctor or laboratory technician will draw a tube of blood from your arm, then give you a drink of quickly absorbed glucose. This must be swallowed within five minutes. An hour later another blood sample is drawn, followed by samples taken at two hours and three hours (and sometimes at four and five hours). The glucose content of each blood sample is carefully measured. (NOTE: Many doctors take a blood sample in the first half hour following the glucose intake. This provides no information useful for diagnostic purposes.)

## WHAT THE BLOOD TELLS US

The glucose tolerance test gives readings of blood sugar for at least four different time periods—fasting, one hour, two hours, three hours. These are plotted into a curve and analyzed.

For the normal person without diabetes or hypoglycemia, blood sugar throughout the day will be between 0.070 and 0.2 grams per 100 cc of blood. In other words, whether or not the patient has recently had a meal, there is always approximately 7 to 20 parts sugar to one hundred parts of blood. A blood value of 70 to 100 mgs percent corresponds to a blood *serum* level of 115 mgs percent. The serum, the fluid left after the blood cells and blood-clotting substances are removed, is what is tested in most chemical determinations today.

By the way, the numbers you get with a home finger-stick blood test are usually lower than the readings from a laboratory because at home you are measuring whole blood, which has a lower sugar content for the same volume than serum alone.

In the normal person, the serum level rises an hour after eating to no more than 175 mgs percent (up to 200 mgs is still considered normal), and at two hours drops back to no more than 145 mgs percent. At three hours, it returns to the fasting level.

But, if you are a diabetic, your numbers will be different. When your fasting level is above 126 mgs, your one-hour level above 175 mgs, two-hour level above 145, and three-hour level above 126, you have abnormally elevated glucose and you have confirmed diabetes.

Sometimes a diagnosis is made when three out of the four tests on the curve show elevated glucose, and sometimes a system of totaling the numbers is used. When the fasting, one-hour, two-hour, and three-hour results are added together and produce a sum below 500, you are considered normal. From 500 to 800, you may be diabetic. With a total over 800, you are definitely diabetic.

Treatment—diet alone, or diet plus oral agents or insulin— is necessary if you have the symptoms of diabetes as well as abnormal sugars, or if you have no symptoms but have a fasting sugar over 126 and a two-hour sugar over 200.

The following chart gives examples of representative glucose tolerance tests:

TYPICAL GLUCOSE TOLERANCE TEST RESULTS

|  | *Fasting* | *1 hour* | *2 hours* | *3 hours* | *4 hours* | *5 hours* |
|---|---|---|---|---|---|---|
| Normal glucose | 80 mgs | 125 mgs | 90 mgs | 86 mgs | 84 mgs | 86 mgs |
| Type 2 Diabetic (NIDDM) | 150 | 230 | 210 | 150 | 118 | — |
| Type 1 Diabetic (IDDM) | 250 | 440 | 300 | 280 | 250 | 200 |
| Nonorganic Reactive Hypoglycemic | 90 | 180 | 110 | 100 | 40 | 60 |

## THE LATEST GUIDELINES FOR DIABETES DIAGNOSIS

In 1997, the blood-sugar levels traditionally used to diagnose diabetes were reviewed and revised downward by the American Diabetes Association and endorsed by federal health authorities. Until that time, a blood-sugar level below 140 mgs percent was considered normal. Now, if you have a sugar level over 126 milligrams per deciliter, in two readings, on two different days, on a fasting plasma glucose test, you are classified as diabetic.

The new criteria were developed after it was shown that 10 to 20 percent of diabetic patients develop complications such as eye, kidney, and blood-vessel damage by the time their glucose level reaches 140 mgs percent. With earlier detection and treatment, these complications could be delayed or even prevented.

Here are the new numbers:

A normal fasting blood-sugar level is 104 mgs percent or less. Impaired glucose tolerance, or IGT (see page 30), is defined as 104 to 126 mgs percent. And diabetes is confirmed with blood sugar over 126 mgs percent.

At two hours after eating, 140 mgs percent or less is deemed normal; 140 to 199 mgs is impaired glucose tolerance; 200 mgs percent or higher is classified as diabetes.

## HIGH SUGAR AND YOUR HEART

In a study of almost 7,000 healthy men, ages forty-four to fifty-five, enrolled in the Paris Prospective Study from 1968 and 1973 and followed up for twenty-three years, it was found that the death rate from coronary heart disease almost doubled among those volunteers with fasting blood sugars consistently over 124 mgs. The rate tripled for the men with sugars over 140.

Translation: the higher your sugar level, the higher your chances of developing heart disease.

## IMPAIRED GLUCOSE TOLERANCE

Sometimes blood tests indicate a diagnosis not of diabetes but of impaired glucose tolerance (IGT). This means your blood-sugar levels are higher than normal but not high enough to be considered diabetes. Your measurements fall somewhere between those of the normal person and the diabetic, perhaps with blood sugar becoming abnormally elevated in response to glucose, then returning almost to normal after three hours.

If you have IGT, you do not have diabetes. On the other hand, you may well develop it later because IGT is a major risk factor for type 2 diabetes. Seven percent of those with confirmed impaired tolerance convert to diabetes every year and half eventually end up with the disease. So people diagnosed with IGT should go to the doctor frequently for blood tests and read Chapter 17 for ways to minimize their risk.

# 4

# NOBODY LOVES
# A DIET

Ask 100 people to tell you the secret of diabetes control and 99 of them will answer "insulin." They are wrong. The real secret lies not in that little white bottle, or even in small white, blue, or yellow pills, but in your refrigerator and kitchen cabinets. That fact is not glamorous, mysterious, or even very interesting, but it is true.

What you eat—your diet—is the single most important key to diabetic control. It is the best blood-sugar-lowering agent, the most effective and the least expensive. With diet, plus a certain amount of physical activity, you may not need insulin or oral antidiabetic agents at all. The vast majority of diabetics (and most hypoglycemics) can be controlled with diet alone. Many diabetics who now take oral agents or insulin won't need them anymore if they eat correctly. And some who are overweight will lose all their diabetic symptoms *completely* simply by taking off a few pounds.

As for those diabetics who have truly deficient pancreases and therefore require insulin injections to supply their bodies with this essential hormone, and those who can never utilize their own insulin efficiently without the help of oral agents, diet is *still* the most important ingredient of treatment. Diabetics can never achieve good control, with or without medication, unless they eat correctly.

Nobody loves a diet. Diets tell you not to eat this, and that you must eat that—no fun at all. Most people, when they are first diagnosed as diabetics, are concerned about the need to change their eating habits. After all, the majority of diabetics are overweight and they love food. They don't want to think about every bite that goes into their mouths.

But we are going to make it simple by prescribing what we believe to be the world's easiest and most effective diet. Never have diabetics (or hypoglycemics) had to think less about their food than with this plan. And yet it works.

This diet is not concerned with calories (unless, of course, you want to lose weight). It is concerned only with carbohydrates. *You must eat a certain number of grams of carbohydrates (though not refined sugar) at every meal. That is the only rule. Aside from that, you can eat anything you like if your weight is where you want it to be.*

The diet presented here will not make you miserable, frustrated, or confused. It will keep your blood sugar within the normal range that is now your chief goal. It is safe. It can be followed for a lifetime without difficulty. It is good not only for you, but for the rest of the family as well, so you won't require separate preparation of meals. As you can see, with only a little caution you can eat just like the rest of the world.

## THE CHANGING SCENE IN DIABETIC DIETS

Before the discovery of insulin in 1922, a harsh dietary regimen was the only treatment for diabetes. It usually included very little carbohydrate because once the blood sugar went up it would take off like a runaway train, precipitating a hasty demise as a result of diabetic coma. Diabetics were placed on starvation diets so low in calories that growth was retarded and they died of malnutrition if not diabetic complications; or they were given diets that included only milk and barley water boiled with bread; or rancid meats, fat, and milk served up with lime water, cathartics, and opium; or fat combined with alcohol and vegetables boiled three times before they could be eaten. One nineteenth-century physician made sure his patients ate exactly what he prescribed by locking them in their rooms and opening their doors only to offer them their meager food.

Once insulin was discovered, many doctors decided that patients taking injections could eat whatever they liked, which proved to be a mistake. Others still insisted that carbohydrates be kept low, perhaps to about 30 percent of the daily intake, with the major part of the calories made up of protein and fat.

Recently, however, it has been recognized that diabetics— who already have an accelerated tendency toward arterioslerosis, heart attacks, and strokes—were hastened along the road to vascular disease by the high-fat diet. The diet, in other words, was probably killing more people than it helped. In the early seventies, the American Diabetes Association recommended that diabetics eat the same proportion of carbohydrates as most other people do—50 percent or more.

But even with the liberalizing of the diet, many people continue to find it extremely difficult to stay with a plan that is rigid or complicated. The diet you'll find here is easy to live with, simple, rational, logical. Besides, it works wherever you are. You can follow it to achieve blood-sugar levels within normal boundaries whether you eat at home, in restaurants, or traveling around the world.

## THE WORLD'S EASIEST DIABETIC DIET

To follow this diet, there is just one rule: *avoid simple carbohydrates such as sugar, honey, and syrups* (see page 38) *and eat 40 to 50 grams of complex carbohydrates at every meal.* (Exception: If you are engaging in strenuous exercise, you may need more.)

Forty to 50 grams of carbohydrate amounts to 50 to 60 percent of your daily food, approximating the typical American diet. The rest of your menu will include protein, fats, and water in whatever proportions you choose. If you are not trying to reduce, you may eat as much of these foods as you wish. If you are, you can control your calories up or down simply by adjusting your meat portions. Or, if you prefer, you may incorporate the food exchange lists of the American Diabetes Association to help you keep your calories counted.

Most diets designed for diabetics not only place great emphasis on cutting back carbohydrates (usually cutting them back too much), but also regulate the amount of proteins and fats you can eat at each meal. However, unless you are among the very small number of people whose control is very precarious (there are some slim people who are uncontrolled on diet or oral agents who, with a restricted calorie diet, may avoid insulin) or you are trying to lose weight, there is no need to be concerned about anything but your carbohydrate intake. You will probably consume about the same amounts of proteins and fats every day anyway, and even if you stray from your usual habits one day it won't disturb your blood sugar enough to cause problems when you are in good control. So, simply keep tabs on your carbohydrates. And relax!

## THE COMPONENTS OF FOOD

All foods are made up of carbohydrate, protein, or fat, plus water, minerals, vitamins, and fiber.

*Carbohydrates* (found mainly in sugar, starch, fruits, and vegetables) are the natural fuel of the body and supply the energy to run all its complicated systems. If there is a shortage of carbohydrates in your diet, you will start burning fat, which, in a diabetic, can lead to serious complications. Together with protein and fats, carbohydrates promote the growth and maintenance of body cells. Every gram of carbohydrate is equal to 4 calories.

*Proteins* are the building blocks of the body, needed for growth and repair of body tissues. Most protein foods (chiefly meat, milk, cheese, eggs, fish) contain a large proportion of fat as well. Approximately 58 percent of the protein we eat is slowly converted to carbohydrate. Each gram of protein is equal to 4 calories.

*Fats* provide a concentrated source of energy and add flavor to foods. They carry vitamins along with essential fatty acids, and provide cushioning for vital organs. Each gram of fat equals 9 calories. About 10 percent of the fat we eat is converted to carbohydrate.

*Water* is needed for all the digestive processes and is an essential part of all tissues.

*Minerals and iron* promote strong bones and teeth, healthy circulatory, muscular, and nervous systems, blood hemoglobin, etc.

*Vitamins* are essential for the proper functioning of all systems of the body.

*Fiber* (or roughage) is not a nutrient, but important for efficient digestion and, it is thought, helps maintain normal blood-sugar levels.

## WHAT IS A CALORIE?

A calorie is the amount of energy required to raise the temperature of four gallons of water one degree Farenheit. Another way of putting it is that it is the energy expended by a seated man turning a doorknob.

Though most diets are based on calorie-counting, we are not concerned here with calories—unless, of course, you want to lose weight. Then calories definitely do count because weight cannot be lost (except *temporarily* through water loss on high-protein diets) without cutting calories.

## WHY THINK ABOUT GRAMS?

It's all a numbers game. Our diet uses grams as the basic weight measurement of food. Why? Because grams are much easier to count and manipulate than ounces and pounds, and much more exact. (One pound equals 456 grams, while 1 ounce equals 30 grams. A nickel weighs 5 grams.)

It is essential for our diet to know the number of grams of carbohydrate in each food. That's because we must know how much of that food will enter the bloodstream in the form of sugar, and how quickly it will be absorbed. A diabetic or hypoglycemic can safely handle only a certain amount of sugar at one time. Too much too fast will raise a diabetic's blood sugar too high, and cause a hypoglycemic's blood sugar to rebound too low.

Every food can be analyzed into grams of carbohydrate, protein, and fat. For example, a standard slice of bread weighs about one ounce, or 30 grams. This slice of bread contains 15 grams of carbohydrate, 2½ grams of protein, and 12½ grams of nondigestible material and water.

A small orange weighing 100 grams contains about 10 grams of carbohydrate.

Thirty grams (1 ounce) of meat has no carbohydrate, 7 grams of protein, and 5 grams of fat. The rest is nondigestible material.

## WHY CONCENTRATE ON CARBOHYDRATES?

You must know how much sugar is entering your bloodstream at any one time, because this is the main influence on your blood-sugar level. You require a certain amount, which is derived from carbohydrate, for your brain and body to function, but you cannot cope with too much.

The normal fate of 100 grams of carbohydrate eaten at one sitting is as follows: 25 grams are used by the brain and red blood cells; 60 grams are delivered to the liver to be stored as glycogen for later release or transported into the fatty-acid cycle; the remaining 15 grams are rationed out via the bloodstream to the periphery of the body to be used by the muscles at a rate of 5 grams an hour.

In the nondiabetic, this balance is always maintained by the prompt response of the pancreas to rising blood sugar.

But diabetics are different. Because you produce insufficient insulin or your cells cannot absorb the glucose readily, your blood-sugar levels are not kept at the normal percentage but can rise astronomically when too much carbohydrate is eaten at one time. And they can remain high for a very long time. The excess glucose is excreted along with the urine, or it stays in the bloodstream as elevated blood sugar.

Hypoglycemics are different too. They release *too much* insulin in response to excess sugar, clearing too much glucose from the bloodstream too quickly and so producing very low blood sugar.

## THE NITTY-GRITTY OF CARBOHYDRATES

Carbohydrates contain one or more chains of 3 to 7 carbons, 12 hydrogens, and 6 oxygens, bound together. The smaller the number of chains, the faster they are absorbed by the body. One-chain carbohydrates are monosaccharides, such as glucose, fructose, and galactose. These are absorbed into the bloodstream very quickly.

Oligosaccharides are usually composed of 2 to 4 or more chains of simple sugars, the best known being sucrose found in cane sugar and beets, maltose found in starch, and lactose in milk.

Polysaccharides are long and complex chains of sugar that are the readily digestible storage materials of plant and animal cells. These are starch, dextrin, and glycogen. They are more slowly absorbed and have less immediate effect on blood sugar.

Sorbitol and mannitol are "sugar alcohols," frequently ingredients of "dietetic" foods. They are absorbed slowly and the small amounts in sugarless gum or mints don't add up to enough to affect your blood sugar unless, of course, you eat too much of them. You'd find that 12 pieces of sorbitol-sweetened hard candy, for example, would affect your blood sugar. Besides, 12 pieces would contain 150 calories and could cause diarrhea.

## WHAT YOU CAN'T EAT

Foods that contain simple carbohydrates or sugars—the monosaccharides—must be avoided except upon rare occasions. They contain many calories but very little nutrition. More important, they are *much* too quickly absorbed by the bloodstream. They are too potent. They are available too soon, too precipitously, to be effectively handled by diabetics, especially if you take insulin. They are *dangerous* for you (except when you *need* them to raise your blood sugar in a hurry). DO NOT EAT THEM.

Foods containing simple carbohydrates or sugars include:

Candy
Cereals that are sugar-coated
    or contain sweetening
Condensed milk
Dried fruits
Honey
Jams and jellies
Marmalade and preserves
Molasses
Pastries and cookies
Puddings, pies, and cakes
Raisins
Regular chewing gum
Regular soft drinks
Sugar, any variety, any color
Sweet wine
Syrups

Other foods that diabetics and most hypoglycemics should avoid because they raise blood-sugar levels far too fast are:

Apple juice
Apples
Gelatin desserts (regular)
Grape juice
Instant breakfasts or
    "diet" bars
Maple-sugar-flavored bacon
    or sausage
Pineapple
Pineapple juice
Processed yogurt with fruit
    or flavoring (most brands)
Prune juice
Sherbet
Yams and sweet potatoes

Sometimes you can be surprised by the foods that tend to raise your blood sugar too fast. For example, some people can tolerate ice cream more easily than potatoes. Dietetic pies may be made without added sugar but the fruit in them contains sugar and their crusts must be counted as carbohydrates. Even sugar-free jams and jellies contain natural sugars. An occasional smear isn't a problem but in normal amounts they raise your blood sugar too much.

There has been a lot of talk about the "glycemic index," which means that some foods have more effect on your blood sugar than others even though they may be equivalent in carbohydrate content. You can determine what your glycemic index is for particular foods by testing your blood after you eat them, taking into account the other foods eaten in the same meal. If you find that a food sends your blood sugar way up, avoid it or simply eat less of it.

## IS SUGAR ABSOLUTELY OFF-LIMITS?

Diabetics have long been told to stay away from sugar and sugar-laden foods because simple carbohydrates cause a sudden surge in blood glucose levels, and we are telling you that very same thing again right here. Despite what you may have been reading recently, simple sugars are more quickly absorbed into the bloodstream than other carbohydrates such as starches or complex carbohydrates.

If you yearn for something sweet, it won't hurt you to substitute a cookie or two, a piece of pound cake, or a scoop of ice cream once in a great while for an *equal* amount of carbohydrate in your meal plan. Just remember, however, that you're not getting the same nutrition from a cookie as, say, an orange. And a chocolate peanut chew is certainly not better for you than a couple of slices of bread unless at that very moment you are overdosing on insulin.

## WHAT YOU CAN EAT: THE COMPLEX CARBOHYDRATES

The complex carbohydrates, some of the oligosaccharides and the polysaccharides, are the ones that must make up most of your 40 to 50 grams per meal. They are a much better source of energy than fatty foods because they have less than half the calories of fat and the same amount as protein, and often contain more nutrition in the form of vitamins, minerals, and fiber. Besides, they can make you feel full and more satisfied.

The complex carbohydrates include grains, starches, some vegetables, and legumes. They are absorbed much more slowly than the simple carbohydrates and, eaten in certain amounts, won't raise your blood sugar to abnormal heights that may overwhelm your body. If you stay within the guidelines, your blood sugar should measure no more than 140 mgs percent fasting and 199 mgs percent two hours after a meal—just where we want it.

If you find that this is not true for you, then you must make adjustments in the food you eat. Nothing is chiseled in stone and everything can be changed to suit your special needs.

For your 40 to 50 grams of carbohydrates per meal, choose from the food lists that follow: 10-gram fruits and desserts; 15-gram starches; 3-percent vegetables; 6-percent vegetables.

*Each meal should include no more than 2 units from the 15-gram list* (the equivalent of 2 slices of bread) unless you're about to engage in heavy physical activity, in which case you'll need more. You need this slowly absorbed carbohydrate to carry you over to your next meal or snack. Fruits and juices, because they are so quickly digested and absorbed, raising your blood sugar more rapidly, *cannot be used as most or all of your total allotment.*

Keep your meals well balanced and varied, and eat the rest of your calories in proteins and fats as you like. How much of these you eat is a matter of taste and habit. Most people consume about the same amounts every day or every week. If, however, you are watching your weight or your cholesterol level, then your proteins and fats should be limited as we will discuss a little later.

Diabetics who take insulin must take care to eat the *same* amount of food, including the *right* amount of carbohydrate, every day, spaced out in the *same* way, because your insulin dose is based on the food you consume.

NOTE: You will see that we have included milk and plain yogurt in *both* the 10-gram (fruits) list and the 15-gram (starches) list. Because they are intermediate in both absorption rate and carbohydrate content, you may substitute them for foods on either list. They also contain protein and fat. Avoid the flavored and fruited yogurts. Vanilla yogurt, for example, has twice as much carbohydrate as plain. Some brands of cherry yogurt have almost three times as much. Always check the container for carbohydrate content and figure it into your total amount for that meal.

Tomato sauce is also on two lists, the 10-gram list and the 6-percent vegetable list, because its carbohydrate content falls between the two.

### *Foods containing 10 grams of carbohydrate*

2 medium apricots
½ medium banana
½ cup blueberries, black-
    berries, or raspberries
½ small cantaloupe
9 cherries
¾ cup diet cranberry juice
¼ cup diet cranberry
    sauce
1 medium fresh fig
½ medium grapefruit
5 ounces grapefruit juice
15 grapes
3 medium lemons
½ small mango
⅛ large melon (honeydew)
1 medium nectarine
1 small orange
3 ounces orange juice

1 small peach
1 small pear
2 small plums
2 cups popcorn
1 cup strawberries
1 large tangerine
8 ounces (1 cup) tomato
    juice or 6 ounces
    vegetable juice
½ cup tomato sauce
1 cup watermelon balls
¾ cup plain yogurt

*Also:*
1 scoop ice cream*
1 scoop ice milk*
1 scoop frozen yogurt
½ cup evaporated milk
8 ounces (1 cup) milk†

---

* Vanilla, chocolate, coffee, or strawberry. If you eat dietetic ice cream, you may have ¼ pint, the equivalent of a 10-gram serving.
† Whole, skim, low-fat, buttermilk, or powdered (¼ cup diluted with ¾ cup water).

*Also:*
5 animal crackers
1 "thin" slice of bread
1 slice protein bread
2 fortune cookies
3 gingersnaps
44 thin pretzel sticks
2 graham crackers

2 Lorna Doones
18 oyster crackers
5 Ritz crackers
4 Saltines
3 Social Teas
3 Triscuits
2 Uneeda Biscuits
8 Wheat Thins

### Foods containing 15 grams of carbohydrate

1 slice bread (white, rye, pumpernickel, whole wheat, French, Italian)
1 small plain roll
½ hamburger roll
1 hot-dog roll
½ large pita
½ matzoh
4 small matzoh balls
1 small plain muffin or biscuit
¼ medium bagel
½ plain doughnut
½ English muffin
½ plain croissant
1 slice French toast (without sugar)
1 cheeze blintz
5 thin Melba toasts
3 Zwieback toasts
2 bread sticks
15 potato chips
1 5-inch waffle
1 4-inch pancake
1 small corn muffin
1 8-inch tortilla

2 6-inch taco shells
¼ cup bread crumbs
1 piece marble or pound cake (same weight as 1 slice of bread) on special occasions
3 dietetic chocolate chip cookies

*Also:*
½ cup cooked rice, barley, groats, grits
½ cup cooked macaroni, spaghetti, or other pasta
½ cup cooked egg noodles
1 medium white potato
½ cup mashed potatoes
7½ medium French fries
⅓ cup cooked dry beans (lentil, mung, pinto, red, black, etc.)
¼ cup cooked soybeans
½ small ear corn or ⅓ cup kernels
½ cup cooked cereal
½ cup bran cereal (no raisins)

1 cup puffed cold cereal
¾ cup most other cold
  cereals
2 tbsp. wheat germ (plain)
2 tbsp. miller's bran
1 small California
  avocado or ½ small
  Florida avocado

*Also:*
  8 ounces (1 cup) milk*
  ½ cup evaporated milk
  1 cup plain yogurt

NOTE: Any item from the 10-gram list becomes 15 grams by taking one and a half portions. Be careful, however, when you consume more fruit, because it may be absorbed so quickly that it will raise your blood sugar too high and too fast. The only way to check its effect on you is to make frequent blood tests soon after you've eaten it.

Water-packed canned fruits may be eaten in the same amounts as fresh fruit. For example, remember that two halves of a canned pear equal 1 small pear. Don't eat more.

Beware of soup! Sometimes—especially for people who produce little of their own insulin—a bowl of vegetable, lentil, or bean soup will make their blood sugars soar. That's because when legumes are cooked, their skins are softened and their carbohydrate is made available to be absorbed directly into the bloodstream instead of going through the bowel. Our advice: Stay away from soups you can't see through. Again, you can find out if this applies to you by monitoring your blood sugar soon after you've eaten opaque soup.

Another note: Find out where your avocados come from. A small California avocado usually contains only 6.5 grams of carbohydrate while a small Florida avocado may have up to 13 grams.

## A VERITABLE VARIETY OF VEGETABLES

Vegetables also contain carbohydrate, and it is important to know how much of them you can safely eat. The following

---

* Whole, skim, low-fat, buttermilk, or powdered (¼ cup diluted with ¾ cup water).

list includes those that have only 3 grams of carbohydrate per 100 grams of weight and in most cases influence your blood sugar very little. They consist mainly of water and nondigestible fiber. Eat them raw as you like. If cooked, limit them to about 1 cup per portion.

### 3-percent vegetables

Asparagus, fresh
Bamboo shoots
Bean sprouts
Broccoli
Cabbage
Cauliflower
Celery
Cucumber
Eggplant
Endive
Green or wax beans
Green pepper
Kohlrabi
Lettuce, romaine, chicory, escarole
Mushrooms
Parsley
Radishes
Rhubarb (no sugar)
Sauerkraut
Spinach
Summer squash
Swiss chard
Turnip
Watercress
Zucchini

The 6-percent vegetables have 6 grams of carbohydrate for every 100 grams of weight and cannot be taken ad lib by many diabetics. These are usually restricted to ½ cup per meal (or counted as 5 grams of your total of 40 to 50 grams). If you want to eat more, subtract appropriately from your starch.

### 6-percent vegetables

Artichokes
Brussels sprouts
Carrots
Green peas
Kale
Okra
Onions, leeks, chives, scallions
Pumpkin
Red peppers
Tomatoes
Tomato sauce
Turnips
Winter squash

## THE SECRET OF SUCCESS

The only way you can successfully stick to the 40 to 50 grams per meal of carbohydrate without constantly counting and figuring and going bananas is to remember the equivalents of *two slices of bread!*

Once you can remember that the equivalent (which is how much *complex* carbohydrate you must have every meal—30 grams) is 1 cup of rice or pasta, 2 medium potatoes, 15 French fries, 1 English muffin, ⅔ cup of corn, 1 cup of cooked cereal, etc., you can go anywhere, eat in any restaurant and be perfectly safe. We are assuming you will not only eat your two-slices-of-bread equivalent per meal but another 10 to 20 grams of carbohydrate as well.

Your body cannot distinguish between rice or bread or beans. Or, from the fruit list, it doesn't know the difference between strawberries, grapefruit, or blueberries. It only knows it is getting so many grams of complex or simple carbohydrates. Interchange the foods on each list as you like and your body won't care.

By the way, pasta cooked *al dente* contains more carbohydrate than well-cooked pasta because it has less water content (the longer it cooks, the more water it absorbs), so your portion should be a little smaller. The sauce on your pasta makes a difference as well. Sauces such as garlic and olive oil, primavera, and pesto are acceptable, but watch out for tomato sauce. Tomato sauce raises blood sugar too quickly for most diabetics, especially those on insulin.

## PLANNING YOUR MEALS

To plan meals, there is only one rule: *40 to 50 grams of carbohydrate, with at least 30 grams coming from the starch list.* There's no need to count right down to the very last gram—*approximately* 40 to 50 is sufficient. This makes it very simple. If you can remember the national anthem, you will soon remember the values of the foods you usually eat.

Do not save carbohydrates from one meal to another. Eat your full allotment at each meal or you may run into low-sugar trouble.

Eat about the same number of grams of carbohydrate every day (the only exception: when you plan unusually heavy exercise or nonexercise. See Chapter 5). This is most important for insulin-users, not so critical for those on oral agents, and usually matters not at all if you are diet-controlled. Dosages of insulin are designed to correspond to your food intake. If your carbohydrate intake changes, you will suffer from too much insulin or too little.

Let's start with breakfast.

## Breakfast

We will assume you eat the typical American breakfast, but you may make your own choices as long as you avoid simple sugars and limit yourself to 40 to 50 grams of other carbohydrates. You only need to do your arithmetic.

For example, you might choose one of the following:

- 3 ounces orange juice, 8 ounces tomato juice, or ½ cantaloupe for your breakfast fruit. This accounts for 10 grams of carbohydrate.

Then, adding another 30 grams, choose among these:

- 2 slices toast, 2 halves English muffin, ½ bagel, 2 small corn muffins, 2 4-inch pancakes, or 2 slices of French toast. These are worth 15 grams each or 30 grams in all.
- Coffee or tea.

This meal contains about 40 grams of carbohydrate.

If you prefer cereal, have 1 cup of cold cereal with 8 ounces of milk or 1 cup of hot cereal with 4 ounces of milk.

## Helpful Hints

Sometimes you may want ½ banana on your cereal. Then omit the juice or other fruit or drink only a small glass of tomato juice.

If you'd like to add eggs or bacon or any other protein or fat, feel free. The only reason to restrict them is for weight or cholesterol reduction.

Why can't you eat a whole bagel as your 30 grams of bread? Because a bagel is the equivalent of four slices of bread (60 grams). Your portion is half a bagel, even if you've scooped out some of the middle. Think of it this way: if you threw a bagel at somebody's head you could kill him but if you threw two slices of bread at him he'd laugh. Bagels are dense and heavy—half is all you get.

The small amount of milk you use in coffee or tea needn't be counted.

Coffee and tea present no special problems for the diabetic. Hypoglycemics, however, sometimes do better with decaffeinated beverages.

Artificial sweeteners may be used (unless you are pregnant).

Obviously you won't use real syrup on your pancakes or French toast. Use only tub margarine or add a *little* dietetic syrup or jelly.

If you take insulin, always be sure to eat the same amount of carbohydrate every morning. Your dose of insulin is predicated on the food you eat. When you eat less, you may have a reaction. When you eat more, you may raise your sugar level. Always have the same kind of breakfast with the same combination of starches and proteins.

To help you plan breakfast, here are the carbohydrate values of 1 cup of some popular cereals. Not included are the sugar-coated varieties, which you must not eat. Note that Grape-Nuts are very high in carbohydrate and that the bran cereals are also high. Avoid Grape-Nuts and eat only ½ cup of bran cereal or Wheat Chex for your equivalent of two slices of bread.

| Cereal (1 cup) | Grams of carbohydrate |
| --- | --- |
| All-Bran | 44 |
| Bran Buds | 72 |
| Cheerios | 23 |
| Cornflakes | 24 |

| Cereal (1 cup) | Grams of carbohydrate |
|---|---|
| 40% Bran Flakes | 30 |
| Grape-Nuts | 92 |
| Grapenut Flakes | 31 |
| 100% Bran | 69 |
| Nutrigrain | 32 |
| Puffed Rice | 12.8 |
| Puffed Wheat | 8 |
| Raisin Bran | 47 |
| Rice Krispies | 24 |
| Special K | 22 |
| Shredded Wheat (2 biscuits) | 41 |
| Total | 30 |
| Wheat Chex | 52 |
| Wheaties | 24 |

## Lunch and Dinner

Eat whatever you wish, but try to have a balanced meal. Avoid refined sugars and eat no more than 40 to 50 grams of carbohydrate. Include some vegetables as well as protein, which converts slowly to carbohydrate. If your weight and cholesterol are normal, you may have whatever amount of proteins and fats you are accustomed to eating. If not, see page 51.

*Be sure* that every meal includes the equivalent of two slices of bread; or, in other words, two units of the "big" starches found in the 15-gram list. You will need this slowly absorbed carbohydrate to carry you over until your next meal or snack. If all your carbohydrate is taken in the form of fruit or juices (10-gram list), it may throw your blood sugar into a tailspin. On the other hand, always include as well a selection from the 10-gram list to provide the blood sugar you will need in the next couple of hours.

Your lunch may consist of meat or fish, 2 slices of bread or a starch equivalent, one 3-percent vegetable, one 6-percent vegetable. Plus coffee, tea, or a diet drink. For most insulin-taking diabetics, it's best not to eat fruit at lunch because it can raise your blood sugar too much. The long-acting insulin you've taken in the morning won't peak until about 3 P.M.

For example, perhaps you will choose for lunch
- 3 ounces of meat (0 carbohydrate)
- Salad with lettuce and ½ cup tomatoes (6 grams carbohydrate), with French dressing (1 tablespoon or 3½ grams)
- 2 slices of bread (30 grams)

This adds up to 39½ grams of carbohydrate, right in the ballpark.

For dinner, perhaps you will eat
- 3 to 6 ounces of chicken (0 carbohydrate)
- 1 ear of corn (30 grams)
- ½ cup of peas (6 grams)
- ½ grapefruit (10 grams)

You have a total of 46 grams of carbohydrate. Always include a 10-gram fruit at dinner.

On special occasions, it is permissible to substitute a piece of marble or pound cake for your bread allowance, if the cake weighs the same as a slice of bread.

## Snacks

Diabetics who take insulin (except for Humalog, which is shorter-acting) should always add two or three snacks to their three meals so their blood sugar never sinks too low. Usually, an afternoon and an evening snack are sufficient, but if you tend to get shaky before lunch, add one in the morning. Diabetics on diet alone or oral agents do not need the snacks because they will almost never have too much insulin in their bloodstreams.

Midmorning: About 10:30 (if you have had your breakfast at 7 or 8 A.M.), eat 10 grams of carbohydrate. Perhaps you'll choose 2 graham crackers, or 3 Social Teas, or a small orange, or a glass of milk.

Midafternoon: About 3 or 4 P.M., have another 10 or 15 grams of carbohydrate.

Before bed: Eat 15 grams of carbohydrate *plus* some protein before you go to sleep. The protein will slowly convert to carbohydrate during the night, warding off early-morning insulin reactions. The only exception to this snack is if you've had a very late dinner, leaving you no time for more food.

Suggestions: 1 slice of bread and a slice of cheese; a glass of milk; half a glass of milk with crackers; one fruit and ½ slice of cheese; half a chicken or tuna sandwich; a scoop of ice cream; peanut butter and crackers.

By the way, you don't have to buy packaged snack bars for your snacks. Regular food will do the job and is far less expensive.

NOTE: the carbohydrate content of the snacks is *in addition to* your 40 to 50 grams per meal. Don't save it from your meals.

## NO INSULIN, NO SNACKS!

Scheduled snacks are required for diabetics who take insulin (except Humalog) but, except for 3-percent vegetables, they are not allowed for those who are controlled by diet or oral hypoglycemic agents. What, no snack before bed? That's right.

On the other hand, if that edict is too cruel for you to live with, here's a compromise: Save a fruit or the equivalent of a slice of bread from dinner and have it before you go to bed.

### Free Foods

Along with the 3-percent raw vegetables, these are foods you can eat as you like because they contain very little or no carbohydrate, or they are used in such small amounts as to be insignificant. For example, 1 ounce of soy sauce has only 2.7 grams of carbohydrate.

Bouillon
Celery salt
Cinnamon
Dietetic candy and gum (up
    to 5 pieces a day)
Dietetic gelatin (up to 1 cup
    a day)
Dietetic jams and jellies
Garlic
Herbs and spices
Horseradish
Lemon
Mayonnaise
Mint
Monosodium glutamate
Mustard
Pepper
Saccharine
Sour or unsweetened dill
    pickles
Soy sauce
Sugar-free sodas
Tartar sauce
Vinegar
Worcestershire sauce

## DIET FOR DUMMIES

The diet we've outlined should be easy for almost anybody to follow, but if all else fails, remember these four simple rules:

1. No double starches. If you have bread at a meal, you can't have a potato. If you have corn, you can't have rice. If you have cereal and milk for breakfast, you must not have bread too. One starch per meal is all you're allowed.

2. No opaque soups. Don't eat soup that you can't see through. Stay away from such soups as pea, barley, lentil, and vegetable.

3. No apples or pineapples. Except for very small apples, they have too much carbohydrate for one sitting unless you exercise a lot, are taking enough insulin to cover it, or are only a mild diabetic.

4. No more than two fruits a day. Exception: If you are on insulin, you may have another one as your 3 P.M. snack.

## IF YOU WANT TO LOSE WEIGHT

To turn this easy carbohydrate-counting diabetic diet into a weight-loss diet, all you have to do is limit the amount of proteins and fats you consume. Remember that with weight loss many adult diabetics can "lose" their disease for years, maybe forever. Others can cut down on their insulin or oral-agent requirements. Sometimes the loss of only a few pounds is enough to increase the number of insulin receptors so that your available insulin is now adequate without outside help.

## ARE YOU OVERWEIGHT?

If you are too heavy, it is imperative to shed some pounds, especially if you are an "apple," a person who is fattest around the middle. You can determine whether you need to lose weight by calculating your body mass index (BMI). A BMI of 25 or more raises your risk of diabetes if you don't already have it, and may be what's keeping you diabetic if you do.

Your BMI is your weight divided by your height squared. Follow these rules: First, multiply your weight in pounds by 705. Divide the result by your height in inches, then divide that result by your height in inches again. For example, if you weigh 200 pounds and are 5 feet 8 inches tall: 200 multiplied by 705 equals 141,000; divided by 68 (inches) once, is 2,073; divided by 68 again, is a little over 30. At a body mass index of 30, you are overweight. Try for a BMI of 25 or less.

## RULES FOR DIABETICS ON A DIET

*Do not* cut back on your 40 to 50 grams of carbohydrate per meal or your snacks if you take insulin. These are essential to your health. Besides, they are not nearly so fattening as fats and almost all protein foods (most of which have a high percentage of fat), a fact which continues to amaze people who have heard all their lives that bread and potatoes put on weight. What puts on weight is too many calories. Fats and the majority of protein foods contain many more calories than starches.

To lose weight, eat very little fat (butter, cream, margarine, oil, cream cheese, nuts, etc.) and stay away from fried foods. Limit your meat or fish portion to 3 ounces at lunch and dinner. You will now have (including your allotted carbohydrates) a 1,000-calorie diet. Remember, you must eat enough carbohydrate to provide the body's essential fuel and prevent acidosis, so *do not* lower your allotment. If you wish to lose more slowly, you may eat 3 ounces of meat or fish for lunch and 6 ounces for dinner.

*If you take insulin, you cannot cut your usual calories without adjusting your dose. So, before you go on a diet, discuss it with your doctor. This is very important.*

If you take oral agents, you probably won't require a change in dosage, but talk it over with your doctor before beginning your new regime.

If you are on diet alone, you have no problem.

## WEIGHT LOSS IN A BOTTLE

Many overweight adult diabetics can "lose" their diabetes or cut back on their need for oral agents or insulin simply by getting rid of some of their extra fat. If you would like to do the same but can't seem to do it on your own, consult your physician about drugs that may help you. Use with caution: Some reducing drugs have been found to cause heart damage.

An aid to weight loss may be soon developed as a result of the discovery of a "fat-melting hormone" called leptin. Researchers are now looking for a way to increase the leptin levels in obese people, thereby helping them to shed their excess pounds.

## GET GOING!

It's easier for most people to attack sloth with an exercise program than to attack gluttony by cutting back on food. Besides, exercise is one of the best ways to lose weight as well as keep your diabetes under control, so try to add some vigorous physical activity to your life (see Chapter 5).

Remember, however, that diabetes control is always a balancing act between food intake and energy expenditure. Especially if you take insulin, you must not change your routine without consulting your physician because you may find yourself flat on the gym floor with an insulin reaction.

## DON'T FOOL AROUND WITH THE DOSE

Diabetic teenage girls often skip their insulin injections because they want to lose weight, according to a study at the Hospital for Sick Children in Toronto. Typically, youngsters with diabetes gain about ten pounds when they start taking insulin. Some of them, desperately eager to be thin, decide to skimp on their prescribed dose, thereby putting themselves at risk for diabetic complications. The researchers found 86 percent of girls with eating problems showed early stages of diabetic retinopathy compared to 24 percent of those with normal eating habits.

The moral: whatever your age, never take it upon yourself to skip or reduce your prescribed insulin dose. The results can be disastrous.

## MEAT AND FISH

Here is what 3 ounces (about 217 calories) of meat or fish amounts to:

| | | |
|---|---|---|
| Lean beef: | Hamburger | 1 large patty |
| | Sliced beef | 2 slices, 4" × 4" × ¼" each |
| | Stew | ½ cup meat |
| | Steak | 1 small steak |
| Lamb: | Roast | 2 slices, 3" × 3" × ½" |
| | Chop | 2 ribs |
| | Stew | ½ cup meat |

| Liver: | | 2 slices, 3″ × 3″ × ¼″ |
| --- | --- | --- |
| Pork: | Chop | 1 large chop |
| | Roast | 1 slice, 3″ × 3″ × ¼″ |
| Veal: | Chop | 1 medium chop, ½″ thick |
| | Roast | 1 slice, 3″ × 3″ × ¼″ |
| Chicken: | Broiler | ½ small broiler |
| | Roast | 3 slices, 3″ × 3″ × ¼″, or 1 leg and 1 slice |
| Turkey: | Roast | 2 slices, 4″ × 3″ × ¼″ |
| Fish: | Fresh halibut, cod, salmon, perch, bass, trout | 1 slice, 3″ × 3″ × 1″ |
| | Tuna | ¾ cup (water packed) |

For each ounce of meat, substitutions are:

1 slice American cheese

2 strips bacon

2 ounces creamed cottage cheese

1 medium egg

1 ounce fish

1 tablespoon peanut butter

5 shrimp, oysters, clams, or scallops

## HOW MANY CALORIES DO YOU NEED?

To maintain their weight just where it is, most adults require 10 calories per pound, plus 3 calories per pound for little activity, 5 calories per pound for moderate exertion, and 10 calories per pound for strenuous exertion, every day.

In addition, pregnant women require an additional 300 calories a day and those who are breast-feeding need an extra 500 calories a day.

## WATCH YOUR CHOLESTEROL LEVEL

Diabetics have a tendency to develop abnormally high levels of cholesterol and/or triglycerides, a situation that leads to heart disease and atherosclerosis (hardening of the arteries). If your test results are way up there, it would be extremely wise to make some changes in your diet by limiting your intake of fats, especially the saturated varieties. Your total cholesterol level should be under 200, triglycerides less than 150, and LDL, the undesirable cholesterol, below 130. If, however, your HDL level is high and its ratio to the LDL is good, then there's probably no need to be concerned about a high total number.

As for triglycerides, fats transported by the blood along with the cholesterol, they can be elevated by poor diabetic control, too much alcohol, and/or excessive consumption of sweets.

Diet can often reduce an abnormally high level of cholesterol at least to some degree, so we recommend that you try. It helps to remember that fat has 280 calories an ounce, or 9 per gram—twice the calories of carbohydrate or protein.

Avoid the foods that contain saturated animal fat and are hard, such as cheese or butter. Cut back on fatty meats, eggs, liver, and other organ meats. Though most liquid fats are made from vegetables and are unsaturated, some, such as coconut or palm oil, should be crossed off your list, and others, such as cottonseed oil, limited. Use soft tub margarine. When margarine is hardened into bars, it becomes partially saturated.

Your goal should be to limit your total fat intake to 30 percent, with less than 10 percent coming from saturated fats. Ask yourself how often you eat hot dogs, sausages, fatty meats, cheese, doughnuts, cookies, cakes, pies, oily or creamy dressings, potato chips, butter, hard margarine, eggs, whole milk, and premium ice cream. If the answer is more than occasionally, you need to reform.

Never fry your food. Instead, bake, broil, poach, or steam. Cook with lemon juice, mustard, spices and herbs, garlic, onion, extracts, artificial sweeteners, vinegar, canola or corn oil. When eating out, ask for sauces and dressings on the side, and don't order fried foods.

Many people are lucky because they can eat all the high-cholesterol foods such as meat and eggs they want without affecting their cholesterol levels. They are born with more lipoprotein lipase, the enzyme that keeps their cholesterol under control. If you aren't among the lucky ones and your cholesterol and triglycerides levels are elevated, it is safe for you as a diabetic to take a cholesterol-lowering drug such as Pravachol, Lescol, Zocor, Mevacor, or Lipitor.

## FAST FOODS: SAFE FOR DIABETICS?

In today's hectic world, families no longer eat home-cooked meals every night and lunches are often taken on the run. For this reason, we should all know the carbohydrate values of the ready-to-eat food we may encounter.

Take, for example, hamburgers: A hamburger roll, top and bottom, is the equivalent of 2 slices of bread (30 grams of carbohydrate). The meat within is your protein. Do not overdo the catsup, since 1 tablespoon equals about 4½ grams of carbohydrate. The dressing also contains some sugar, but a small amount won't matter. Skip the French fries unless you are exercising strenuously or doing some heavy manual labor and need the extra grams of carbohydrate (15 French fries equal 30 grams). Forget the cola (except sugarless) and the milk shake. They are not for you.

As for pizza parlors, remember 1 slice of pizza equals almost 2 slices of bread, or 30 grams.

Now let's consider "fish 'n' chips." The batter counts as a bread. Fifteen French fries would be the equivalent of 2 slices of bread. Go easy on the coleslaw because it probably contains sugar.

### More Helpful Hints

• A banana is a banana, whether it is green, yellow, or purple, and contains about the same amount of carbohydrate even if it is called a plantain.

• Fructose is not for you because it is converted very quickly into glucose and raises your blood sugar accordingly. The more diabetic you are—meaning the less natural insulin you have available—the quicker the fructose changes to glucose.

• Apple, pineapple, grape, and prune juices, even unsweetened, are all no-nos because their sugars are much too rapidly absorbed into the bloodstream.

Whole apples, too, frequently affect glucose tolerance adversely and should be avoided by most diabetics and hypoglycemics. A decent-size apple often contains 30 grams of rapidly metabolized sugar.

• For the same reason, stay away from applesauce, even if it is unsweetened. It is loaded with natural sugar.

• It won't help you a bit to toast your bread or eat it stale. It still retains its carbohydrate content and has merely lost its water content.

• Common pitfalls are dried fruits—raisins, prunes, dried figs, pineapple, apricots, etc. They are *very* high in concentrated sugar.

• Go easy on nuts too. A few won't hurt you, but a lot may send your blood sugar sky high. A pregnant woman from Hong Kong was referred to this office because she had developed diabetes. Warning her against the cashews to which she was devoted was all that was necessary. Seven cashews contain as much sugar as a fruit. As for other nuts, 30 pistachios, 22 peanuts, 10 walnuts, or 15 almonds are equal in carbohydrate to half a fruit portion. A couple of nuts won't destroy you, but if you eat more than that, count them as all or part of a fruit.

• Soups frequently are the cause of a blood-sugar disaster. One patient had a very erratic pattern, with reactions one day, high sugars the next, and decided she was a brittle diabetic. It turned out the brittleness was in the soup she was eating. She ate lunch at the same restaurant every day, always ordering the soup of the day. The thick soups—barley, lentil, pea, or minestrone vegetable soups—made her sugar soar. All of these soups contain astonishing concentrations of carbohydrate, too much for one meal. The days she had plain chicken soup were the days she had insulin reactions.

The soups you can eat without worry include: chicken, onion, some tomato soups, mushroom, celery, zucchini, gazpacho, cucumber—the plain soups.

If you eat creamed soup or chowders made with flour, omit one of your two units of starch for that meal. The same applies for heavy gravies.

Borscht, which is made from beets, which are high in sugar, should be crossed off your list.

Miso soup is another one to avoid—a half cup contains 38.6 grams of carbohydrate, the equivalent of more than two slices of bread.

• Remember sugars and simple carbohydrates are often needed to fight off insulin reactions, but the complex carbohydrates plus protein are best if you have time and they work for you.

• When you are planning to get involved in heavy exercise or manual labor, take extra carbohydrates before you begin. Some people need 60 or 70 grams per meal to compensate for strenuous physical activity.

• On the other hand, if you are suddenly not getting your accustomed exercise—if you are in bed with a broken leg— you will require more insulin and maybe less carbohydrate. Only your blood tests will give you the answer.

• Avoid "instant" breakfasts and yogurt containing *anything*. The fruits and flavors that are added are usually sugar-laden.

• A few slices of onion on a hamburger or in a salad won't hurt you, but remember that 5 or 6 pearl (or larger) onions in a stew equals about 8 grams of carbohydrate. Proceed with caution. The same with tomatoes—a big ripe tomato that tastes so good right out of the garden can throw your sugar way off.

## MORE PITFALLS

There are so many sugar traps lurking around that it might be helpful to be aware of a few of the more common pitfalls.

These are foods you may never have suspected of containing inordinate amounts of sugar, but could throw your glucose tolerance for a real loop.

• The most popular brand of catsup contains 29 percent sugar. A tablespoon on your hamburger can be tolerated, though.

• If you use a lot of artificial sweeteners, be aware that one package contains 1 gram of sugar, so 4 to 5 packages throughout the day will add up to a lump of sugar. A patient who drank 25 cups of coffee a day (not a good idea for anyone) added a packet of sweetener to each cup, adding up to the equivalent of five teaspoons of sugar—and wondered why his blood sugar was out of control.

• Many processed foods contain amazing amounts of hidden sugar. Learn to read labels before eating concocted foods.

• Other foods with high sugar content include All-Bran, 100% Bran, Bran Buds, Raisin Bran, Grape-Nuts, and, of course, all sugar-coated cereals.

• Beware of "milk imitations," such as nondairy creamers, fake whipped cream, etc. Most of them contain sugar as well as a long list of chemicals. Always ask for fresh milk for your coffee.

• Never substitute "fruit drinks" for fruit juice. They are not only mostly water, which you can get almost free at home, but they are made with lots of sugar. On the other hand, cranberry juice is always diluted with water, making it a fruit drink, because it is too powerful on its own. The regular "cranberry juice cocktail" contains about 32 grams of sugar per 6 ounces. So the low-calorie version—a 6-ounce portion with only 8.5 grams of sugar—is obviously a better choice for you.

• Always take responsibility for your own food. Even hospital dietitians have been known to serve the wrong foods to diabetics, so you must monitor your food just as you do at home, counting your carbohydrates. For example, apple juice, prune juice, and grape juice are frequently found on the hospital breakfast tray. These may not be bowls of granulated sugar nor are they chocolate cookies, but they are still not right for you because they contain too much quickly absorbed sugar that will surely swamp you, especially when you are sick or not exercising.

Perhaps you'll be offered 8 ounces of orange juice (almost 27 grams of quick sugar) as part of your breakfast. It is doubtful you can handle that amount of quick sugar at one time. Or you may be given too many starches at once—bread, corn, potatoes, all in the same meal, for example—which will far exceed your carbohydrate limits, especially when you are in bed and getting no exercise, and even more especially when you will probably get fruit for dessert and perhaps a 6-percent vegetable. At breakfast, don't eat both a roll and a bowl of cereal with milk—that's too much carbohydrate at one time.

Don't eat foods you know are not right for you, even if they arrive on your tray. Argue every debatable item with your doctor and/or the dietitian. Remember you are not exempt from your usual eating pattern just because you are in the hospital. As a matter of fact, now is the time to watch your food more carefully than usual because your illness may make you especially sensitive to fluctuating blood-sugar levels.

• Cottage cheese, pot cheese, cream cheese, sour cream, and other cheeses, though they are milk products, cannot be substituted for milk or yogurt as part of your carbohydrate allotment, but you can include them in your diet as you wish as a protein. No restrictions unless you wish to lose weight. While milk contains about equal amounts of carbohydrate, protein, and fat, these foods have little carbohydrate compared to their protein and fat.

• Breaded foods count toward your total carbohydrates. Omit the equivalent of 1 slice of bread (15 grams) when you eat them.

• Read labels! Some "health" foods, such as Tofutti, contain honey or other forms of sugar and will raise blood sugar in a hurry.

## SPICING UP YOUR SALAD

• If you use just a tablespoon or two of prepared salad dressings, you can get away with most of them. Check the labels to determine their sugar content. When in doubt, make your own dressing or flavor your salad with wine vinegar or lemon, plus spices. You may add oil unless you are trying to lose weight. It contains no carbohydrate.

To help you, here are the carbohydrate values of a few prepared salad dressings.

| Salad dressing (1 tablespoon) | Grams of carbohydrate |
| --- | --- |
| Caesar | 1.0 |
| French | 3.5 |
| Vinaigrette | 1.4 |
| Italian | 0.7 |
| Red wine vinegar, oil | 4.0 |
| Mayonnaise | 3.5 |
| Russian | 4.5 |

Though most salad dressings do not contain much carbohydrate, they are usually laden with calories, a fact to keep in mind if you are overweight. Most low-calorie dressings contain less (some much less) than 3 grams of carbohydrate per tablespoon, but others have more. Read the labels.

Beware of coleslaw—it may contain a lot of mayonnaise and sugar.

## TIMING YOUR FOOD

If you take insulin, *when* you eat is just as important as *what* you eat. *All* diabetics and hypoglycemics should space out their carbohydrate intake throughout the day so that there won't be high peaks and low valleys in blood-sugar levels. But if you take insulin, you must also worry about reactions.

It's important that you eat at specified times because, like a time bomb, the hormone acts at fixed hours of the day. If you don't have food in anticipation of these periods of high insulin action, you will have reactions. You have more flexibility if your regime calls for NPH insulin at night and Regular insulin just before meals. This is a big help to one patient who is an actor and never knows when he'll get a chance to eat a meal.

Never skip a meal or a planned snack. Do not delay your meals. If you are going to a party and know dinner will be served later than your usual mealtime, eat 30 grams of your carbohydrate at your usual time. Then, when you get to the dinner party, skip those 30 grams of carbohydrate (rolls, potatoes, pilaf, etc.) and eat the main course, salad, vegetables, and fruit for dessert. Do not take a chance that you may last until your hostess or the restaurant serves you. Plan ahead or you'll spoil the whole affair for everyone.

## HOW TO BE A HAPPY DINER

Once you know the general rules of diet for a diabetic, then you can apply your common sense when you're eating out. For example, you go to a Chinese restaurant and start with an egg roll. The coating on the egg roll is roughly equivalent to a slice of bread (15 grams of carbohydrate). Now eat a simple main dish, perhaps fish or meat with vegetables, and you can still have the equivalent of another slice of bread. That means a ½ cup of rice or noodles. The carbohydrate value of Chinese soups is negligible if you avoid those containing sugar, such as sweet and sour soup. If you have wonton soup, count three wontons as one bread. Don't eat the duck sauce. Avoid sweet sauces. But have a fortune cookie for good luck!

Using the same common sense, you can eat without fear in any restaurant. When you're out for an Italian dinner, consider a small order of spaghetti to be roughly equal to 2 slices of bread and a fruit. Skip the bread and the bread sticks (two bread sticks equal one bread). Eat the main course and a salad. Italian soups can be a problem because they usually have too much carbohydrate for you. If you skip your two breads and a fruit, you can have two cups of cooked pasta with olive oil and garlic, or pesto, clams, or primavera. But not tomato sauce, which is too high in quickly absorbed sugar. Forget dessert.

At a Middle Eastern restaurant, a regular-size pita counts as two breads. Tabbouleh is a starch just like rice. Shish kebab is no problem. Chick peas, hummus, fava beans, and spinach pies are all heavy starch. Go easy.

Don't order sukiyaki in a Japanese restaurant because it includes questionable amounts of sugar and/or sweet wine. Count the batter coating as a bread exchange when eating tempura. Stay with the simple dishes such as mizutaki—beef or chicken chunks cooked in broth. And remember what we said about miso soup—skip it.


## TO FAST OR NOT TO FAST

Religious fast days such as Yom Kippur can complicate the lives of diabetics who take insulin. If you are controlled by diet alone, fasting is no problem. If you take oral drugs, it is no problem either, but it might be best to skip your pill in the morning and take it before the evening meal that breaks the fast.

For insulin users, fasting is much trickier, and in most cases you would be wise not to try it. Surely your need for food when you are diabetic will not alter the effectiveness of your prayers. It might be better to bend the traditional rules than to encounter a medical emergency.

If fasting is very important to you, however, it can be done. Suppose you normally take 10 Regular and 30 units of Intermediate insulin in the morning. If today is a fast day, take no insulin in the morning, have no breakfast or lunch. Suppose the day goes by and you remain asymptomatic. Check your blood before dinner. If you find you have high sugar (almost a sure bet), do *not* take your usual morning dose. Take more Regular than usual (to compensate for the higher-than-normal sugar) and less Intermediate (because you don't want it to last through the next day). For example: 20 Regular and 20 Intermediate.

But suppose, without insulin, breakfast, and lunch, you begin having symptoms of high sugar and acidosis—frequent urination, thirst, etc. *Do not wait* for dinner. Break the fast *immediately*. Start eating and take your insulin, again increasing your Regular to take care of the high sugar and cutting back on your Intermediate insulin.

Do not do any of the above without consulting your own doctor!

## COMMENTS ON "CHEATING"

There are very few perfect people in this world, and diabetics are no more likely to be among them than anyone else. It is a rare diabetic who doesn't cheat on his prescribed diet once in a while. This is not the end of the world and you shouldn't feel too guilty about it. But it is *not* a good idea to fall off your diet regularly because, if you do, your control will automatically be poor and you will be subject to all the ills and complications that befall poorly controlled diabetics.

For insulin-taking people who cheat occasionally, it is possible to compensate for a binge by taking a blood test after the event and taking a few extra units of Regular insulin if you see very high sugar.

The best way to cheat, however, is to do your forbidden eating before you set off on a program of strenuous exercise, when you may need extra carbohydrates anyway. For example, if you are going to the movies, don't overindulge at dinner. But if your plans include a lot of vigorous dancing, you can probably plan on burning off the excess carbohydrate before the night is out.

## FIBER DIETS: GOOD FOR DIABETICS

According to research, increased fiber in your diet can improve your glucose tolerance. Some fiber foods, such as pectin, guar, and oat bran, are water-soluble. They delay absorption of carbohydrates by trapping them within themselves and releasing them slowly. Because of the delay, less sugar enters the bloodstream immediately after a meal, avoiding an overload. This kind of fiber also seems to lower the level of cholesterol in the blood.

Other fibers, such as cellulose, lignin, and wheat bran, are not water-soluble. They pass through the digestive system quickly, taking other foods along with them, giving the intestines less opportunity to absorb carbohydrates. These also soften the stool and add bulk to it. They have also been shown to help prevent colon cancer.

The canes, roots, and tubers that, before we became so civilized, once constituted the major part of mankind's daily food have been replaced by a diet high in animal proteins and fats as well as grain cereals that have lost most of their fiber content in the milling process. The typical Western diet includes only about four grams of crude fiber a day. In some less-developed countries it makes up thirty grams of the daily diet, and is associated with lower incidences of diabetes, diverticulitis, appendicitis, hemorrhoids, and cancer of the colon. On the other hand, except for lignin found in strawberries and pears, it increases flatulence (gas).

Fiber is indigestible, unabsorbable plant material and is not found in meat or fish. It leaves the digestive system in much the same form it went in and has virtually no caloric value. Nevertheless, it plays a number of vital roles in the digestive process. It is found chiefly in whole grains, nuts and beans, fruits, and vegetables, especially those with edible skins and seeds. It does not matter whether these foods are eaten raw, cooked, frozen, or canned.

Should you, a diabetic, eat a high-fiber diet? More fiber, especially grains, certainly will not hurt you and may well give you an extra little edge. It won't cure your diabetes, but it could tip the scales in your favor. In fact, a large and respected Harvard study of 65,000 healthy women showed that those who ate lots of fiber-rich whole grains—especially in breakfast cereals—had a 28 percent lower risk of developing type 2 diabetes. Eating a high-fiber diet is protective because the fiber slows the absorption of carbohydrates, preventing glucose and insulin from rising steeply. Besides, whole grains contain a variety of nutrients that may boost the body's sensitivity to insulin.

If you are on diet alone or oral agents, you may find that your available insulin is more effective with more fiber. And if you take insulin you may require a little less of the medication. Fiber isn't, however, a cure-all; there is a limit to the amount of it you can eat safely, because most fiber foods are high-starch compounds that take time to be broken down but nonetheless are absorbed as carbohydrate at some time during their metabolism. Among the fiber foods, peas and baked beans have been found to raise blood sugar more than the others.

Important: Remember to include the fiber foods in your 40 to 50 grams of carbohydrate per meal. Dried beans and bran cereals, for example, tend to be high-carbohydrate foods. Two tablespoons of bran or wheat germ equal about 15 grams of carbohydrate, and you must account for it in your total allotment. Sprinkled over a low-carbohydrate cereal (1 cup, or 24 grams), you now have 30 grams. Add a glass of milk, and your total is about 51 grams of carbohydrate, leaving you no more room for carbohydrates at that particular meal.

To get more fiber into your diet, you should eat:

• Whole-grain breads and cereals, especially whole bran or bran-containing foods, or guar, a substance made from the cluster bean and available in health food stores.

• Nuts and seeds. Remember, however, their high carbohydrate content.

• Vegetables such as artichokes, broccoli, cabbage, cauliflower, Brussels sprouts, corn, peas, peppers, beans, cucumbers, carrots.

• Fruits such as strawberries, blueberries, grapefruit, and raw pears.

• Leguminous dried beans—butter, haricot, kidney, soy, lentils, black-eyed, or chick peas, etc. Be careful, however. Beans are high in carbohydrates.

"Fiber breads" may be added to the list. Check the carbohydrate content of each slice so you can be sure to eat a sufficient number of grams.

Caution: Sometimes the absorption of some important trace minerals, such as calcium, zinc, iron, and magnesium, is inhibited when you consume too much fiber. Their absorption, along with that of glucose, may be decreased. So don't go overboard. Eat well-balanced meals that happen to include sufficient fiber.

Some people prefer to get their extra fiber by sprinkling bran into their food. Fruits and vegetables are a much more nutritious alternative, and it is best to get your fiber the natural way, by eating properly. Remember, too, that two flat tablespoons of bran is the equivalent of a slice of bread.

If you are not accustomed to much fiber in your diet, work up to a higher amount gradually. If you notice too much gas or bloating, cut back until you have adjusted. Your body probably will become accustomed to it in a few weeks.

Don't eat your fiber between meals, or it won't have food to act upon. Eat it with your other food.

## DO YOU NEED VITAMINS OR OTHER SUPPLEMENTS?

This is an age of megavitamins, and controversy continues over the need for vitamins and minerals in addition to a balanced diet. Though most medical experts do not think anyone who eats a wide variety of nourishing foods requires supplements, there is some thought that a few of them may be helpful to diabetics. Let's go down the list.

*Vitamin B₁:* This is a vitamin I recommend to my patients with diabetic neuropathy (pain or burning) and about 80 percent of them show some improvement or even complete relief when they take it regularly in daily 100 mg doses. It is especially helpful for neuropathy of the feet. Sometimes injections of up to 20 units of vitamin $B_{12}$ also help.

*Vitamin $B_6$:* Because this is thought to increase glucose tolerance in pregnant women, a supplement of 25 mgs a day is recommended during pregnancy.

*Vitamin C:* Though there is no real scientific proof that it is so, it has been proclaimed that large doses of vitamin C are effective in fighting off numerous ailments, including colds. Many doctors recommend C supplements because they believe it strengthens the capillary walls of the eyes and prevents diabetic eye changes.

We recommend you add 500 mgs of vitamin C to your daily menu.

*Vitamin D,* which comes from sunlight and milk, is thought to improve your ability to rid yourself of glucose and blood fats, metabolize calcium, and keep your blood pressure under control. Be sure to get enough of it. Ten minutes a day in the sun will probably give you an ample supply but just to be sure, take a daily multivitamin supplement that includes 400 I.U. of this important vitamin.

*Vitamin E:* Once known as a vitamin in search of a disease, vitamin E has proved to be an exceedingly valuable nutrient. An antioxidant that is protective against cancer, atherosclerosis, and a substance called PKC-B that is harmful to the artery linings, it also seems to prevent or slow the progression of cataracts, macular degeneration, and diabetic retinopathy, according to a study by the Joslin Diabetes Center in Boston. For all these reasons, we recommend that you take up to 1,000 I.U. of vitamin E every single day.

Don't forget that wheat germ, a favorite source of vitamin E, adds a lot of carbohydrate and must be accounted for in your diet. Two tablespoons count as 15 grams (1 starch).

*Chromium picolinate* has become one of the hot dietary supplements, especially for diabetics. Among the wonders attributed to this natural trace mineral are that it lowers blood sugar, reduces body fat, causes weight loss without dieting, controls appetite, and reduces cholesterol. However, there is still little solid scientific evidence to support any of these claims, except for the few people who are chromium deficient. In addition, high levels of chromium have been associated with cancer and iron deficiency. As a dietary supplement it does not require F.D.A. evaluation or approval.

Having said all that, it remains a possibility that chromium may give your insulin supply a boost. It probably won't hurt you in daily doses of 50 to 200 micrograms from foods such as fruits and vegetables (most Americans consume about 30 micrograms a day) and/or supplements. Talk to your doctor before deciding to take it, however.

*Selenium* is another nutrient that's moving quickly off the shelves today because of its apparent ability to raise blood levels of HDL, the desirable cholesterol, which helps protect against heart disease. However, while the promise of benefit from a daily supplement is strong, it has not yet been proved and most people get plenty of selenium from their food. Major sources include egg yolks, poultry, seafood, whole grains, and foods grown in selenium-rich soil. But because diabetics have blood vessels that can use all the help they can get, it's a good idea to take a daily supplement of 50 to 100 micrograms—if, of course, your own doctor approves.

*Calcium* supplements are recommended for anyone who does not drink much milk, eat a lot of milk products, or get regular exercise. Be sure to consume at least 1,000 mg of calcium a day; 1,500 if you are a postmenopausal woman who does not take estrogen replacement.

*Magnesium* is in short supply in some diabetics with severe retinopathy, but it is not yet known whether adding magnesium salts to your diet will prevent eye changes. A study done in the U.K., however, found that it increased insulin sensitivity in nonobese diabetics. Natural sources: cereals, nuts, beans, meats.

*Zinc* is required for normal growth and development, and some research has shown that, given orally in 200 mg doses, it helps heal diabetic ulcers. It is found naturally in green leafy vegetables, fruits, whole-grain breads, and meat. Don't overdose yourself—too much zinc will cause nausea.

*Vanadium,* a substance that occurs naturally in plants and animals, appears to mimic the action of insulin, speeding up glucose metabolism and decreasing insulin requirements in diabetic animals. In a study at the Joslin Diabetes Center, vanadium improved the glucose tolerance of a series of patients. The safe dose has not yet been determined, however, so, as always, consult your physician before taking it.

*DHEA,* a hormone secreted by the adrenal glands and converted into small amounts of testosterone and estrogen, is claimed to combat everything from aging to obesity to AIDS. Some research suggests that it may improve insulin sensitivity but we urge you not to take it until controlled human studies are conducted and more is known about its long-term safety. As a "dietary supplement" like chromium picolinate and melatonin, it does not require F.D.A. approval, which means its safety and effectiveness have not been scientifically evaluated and nobody knows if it is safe or what the proper dose should be.

*Melatonin* sold in health-food stores is a synthetic version of a human hormone and may help you sleep or overcome jet lag, but probably does little else. We recommend that you stay away from it because serious questions remain regarding proper dosage, interactions with other drugs, and long-term side effects.

NOTE: There is no difference, except in the price, between natural and synthetic vitamins.

## SWEETENERS: BLESSING OR DANGER?

Artificial sweeteners make life a little bit sweeter for people who can't eat sugar, and, from what we know now, there is no reason not to use them, at least in small amounts. A few years ago, experiments with rats showed an increased incidence of bladder tumors among second-generation rats fed the equivalent of 800 saccharin-sweetened diet sodas a day. Saccharin was promptly removed from many homes and hospitals as a result. However, subsequent research on people has completely failed to show the correlation between the sweetener and cancer. Saccharin is now available in many brands, including Sweet'n Low, Sweet Magic, Sugar Twin, Sucaryl, etc.

As for aspartame (Nutrasweet, Equal, Sweetmate, NutraTaste, etc.), it has been approved by the F.D.A. though its safety is still questioned in pregnancy.

It is always best for pregnant women to avoid any artificial chemicals or unnecessary drugs on the chance that they may have an adverse effect on the developing fetus, so they should not use sweeteners. For other diabetics and hypoglycemics, however, they are a much better choice than sugar and keep you from feeling like second-class citizens. Children, especially, need to feel they are not being totally deprived of the goodies their friends consume so freely.

## THE LURE OF "DIETETIC" FOODS

Just because a packaged food (usually very expensive) is labeled "dietetic," it does not mean it is good for diabetics. Although no refined sugar has been included, it may still contain much more carbohydrate than you can handle. Take, for example, dietetic apple pie. Though it may be sweetened artificially, it still has a crust and plenty of apples, and you can exceed your limit without added sugar. On the other hand, you may be able to get away with a piece of dietetic blueberry pie occasionally because it contains a lower sugar content than apple pie, and the natural sugar is not as quickly absorbed. Count the crust as two slices of bread or 30 grams of carbohydrate, and substitute the blueberries for your fruit at dinner. Guide yourself by your blood tests.

Though such items as water-packed canned fruits, dietetic jellies, and gelatin desserts can perk up your menu, many modified foods still contain too much sugar, honey, or syrup for you (though perhaps in smaller amounts than the usual recipe) as well as carbohydrates in other forms.

In general, foods called "noncaloric" or those containing only a few (under 10) calories per serving are safe, eaten in limited amounts. For example, you can safely eat small amounts of dietetic jam or candy. But stay away from dietetic cookies, cakes, chocolates, sherbets, breads, and custards, as well as liquid nondairy creamers, dietetic dinners, and diet bars. Unless you are a chemist, the listed ingredients of most processed dietetic foods are impossible to interpret correctly.

## FAKED OUT BY FRUCTOSE

Once proclaimed to be the answer to a diabetic's dream of a "good" sugar, fructose has not lived up to its expectations. Though this kind of sugar does not require insulin for its metabolism, it converts to glucose in the body and can raise blood-sugar levels just like any of its sugary relatives. The more deficient in insulin you are, the quicker the conversion.

Sorbitol, mannitol, ducitol, and xylitol, all sugar alcohols, are also converted to glucose, but more slowly. You may be able to handle these in tiny amounts, though some people respond to them with cramps and diarrhea.

Avoid carob, a sweetener that tastes like chocolate—it is 75 percent sugar.

## LEARN TO READ LABELS

Sugar comes in many disguises. Beware of any ingredients that end in "-ose" or "-tol." These are usually just plain sugar. For example: dextrose, lactose, sorbitol. Sometimes labels list several varieties of sugar with different names, such as: dextrose, fructose, glucose, sucrose, sorbitol, mannitol, lactose, disaccharide, corn syrup, corn sugar, corn syrup solids, honey, molasses, maltose. Watch out for all of them!

Add a few together in one food and you come up with a high percentage of sugar, more than you can cope with.

Legislation requires that the ingredients of most foods be listed on the label, and also the amounts in grams of carbohydrates, proteins, and fats, according to serving size. Use this information to plan your 40 to 50 grams of carbohydrate per meal.

## NO SMOKING ALLOWED!

We all know by now that smoking is hazardous to everyone's health. For diabetics, who already have a tendency toward vascular disease, smoking is even more dangerous. Smoking affects the coronary blood vessels as well as the smaller vessels in the legs and feet, constricting them, reducing circulation, and affecting the ability of any damaged tissues to heal. In addition, diabetics, especially if they are not in good control, have less oxygen in their tissues than other people. Smoking raises the blood level of carbon monoxide, thus adding to that oxygen deficit. Smoking is also known to increase a tendency toward retinopathy.

If you are a smoker, do yourself an enormous favor and quit.

## MARIJUANA AND OTHER DRUGS

Though there are conflicting reports about the effects of marijuana on mind and body, it is certain that this drug is not a good idea for you. For one thing, it can mask insulin reactions so you may not recognize that you need immediate food. For another thing, it could distort your sense of time so that you may not eat on schedule. And it may set off the "munchies," a craving for sweets that has obvious drawbacks. It may also lower blood pressure in the eyes, a possible prelude to bleeding if you have diabetic retinopathy.

Amphetamines (uppers) are stimulants that can raise or lower your blood sugar unexpectedly. Narcotics (heroin and cocaine) can affect the blood sugar by altering absorption of sugar. So, for these reasons, as well as many others, don't try to get your kicks from drugs.

## GINSENG, A CURE-ALL?

Ginseng, a root popular in Asia, is said to cure many ills, but don't try it if you are diabetic. Ginseng has a steroidlike effect that may raise blood sugar, cause ulcers, and enlarge male breasts, and may well be damaging for anyone.

## ALCOHOL—WHAT DOES IT DO TO YOU?

Being a diabetic (or a hypoglycemic) doesn't mean you must give up all your bad habits. You don't have to go on the wagon and become a teetotaler. On the other hand, you must be a "sensible" drinker. A drink or two a day won't hurt you, if you are in good control and remember a few facts. Actually, alcohol in moderation seems to boost blood levels of high-density lipoproteins (the "good" cholesterol), decrease chances of heart attacks, and inhibit potentially dangerous blood clots. Besides, some studies show that it may increase the body's response to insulin and promote lower blood-sugar levels.

Alcohol has no food value and contains no carbohydrates or other nutrients, though it does add calories to your daily diet. An ounce of whiskey, for example, contains about 85 calories. *Sweet* alcoholic drinks, however, do contain some sugar.

Here are some guidelines to follow:

• Never drink on an empty stomach. Alcohol blocks the process called gluconeogenesis, the formation of glucose from protein and its release from the liver when your blood sugar is too low. Without food, you risk having a severe hypoglycemic reaction if you are on insulin. When you drink before meals, eat some hors d'oeuvres but be sure to count them as part of your meal's allotment of carbohydrate.

• Never have more than two or three ounces of alcohol a day, even with food. You may not be able to recognize an insulin reaction or distinguish it from intoxication. Nor may the police, if you are pulled over for erratic driving. Remember that low blood sugar and intoxication can be—and are—often confused.

• Don't change your insulin dose or diet to allow for your alcoholic drinks.

• Watch out for the "Antabuse effect" if you take Diabinese, an oral hypoglycemic agent. Alcohol will sometimes cause surface blood vessels to dilate, producing marked facial flushing, plus a choking sensation and maybe a headache.

• Sweet drinks do contain carbohydrate. So do the hors d'oeuvres that usually accompany drinking. Avoid sweet wines, stout, cider, ginger beer, port, liqueurs, and cordials. Don't drink sweet mixers such as tonic unless they are sugar-free, and remember that the orange juice in a screwdriver, for example, counts toward your total allotment of quick carbohydrate for that meal. So does Bloody Mary mix (mostly tomato juice).

• A drink before dinner or a glass or two of dry wine with dinner is considered permissible for most diabetics and hypoglycemics. The acceptable list includes: Scotch, rye, whiskey, bourbon, tequila, brandy, rum, gin, sake, vodka, and light dry wine.

• To slip an occasional beer or ale into your life, omit one slice of bread or a fruit at dinner to make up for it. There are about 10 grams of carbohydrate in 8 ounces of regular beer. Some of the "light" beers such as Miller, Schmidt, and Reingold contain only about 3 grams in 8 ounces. Near-beer, such as O'Douls or Sharps, is about the same, but some alcohol-free beers and ales have higher sugar contents, up to 7 grams in 8 ounces, so check them out before you drink them and don't forget to add them to your daily total.

AMOUNTS OF CARBOHYDRATE, ALCOHOL, AND CALORIES IN ALCOHOLIC DRINKS

| Alcoholic Drinks | Amount | Total Grams | Grams of Carbohydrate | Grams of Alcohol | Calories (Approx.) |
|---|---|---|---|---|---|
| Whiskey—Bourbon, Irish, Rye, and Scotch | 1 brandy glass (1 oz.) | 30 | none | 10½–13 | 75–85 |
| Brandy, Gin, Vodka, Sake, Tequila, and Rum | 1 brandy glass (1 oz.) | 30 | none | 10½–13 | 75–90 |
| Liqueurs and Cordials | 1 cordial glass (⅔ oz.) | 20 | 4–10 | 4–7 | 50–80 |
| Malt liquors—ale, beer, porter, and stout | 1 glass (8 oz.) | 240 | 7–14 | 7–14 | 80–150 |
| WINES | | | | | |
| Sweet, domestic | 1 wine glass (3½ oz.) | 100 | 8–14 | 13–15 | 140–165 |
| Sweet, imported | 1 wine glass (3½ oz.) | 100 | 3–20 | 1½–18 | 110–175 |
| *Dry, domestic | 1 wine glass (3½ oz.) | 100 | ½–4 | 10–11 | 75–90 |
| *Dry, imported | 1 wine glass (3½ oz.) | 100 | ½–3 | 8–14 | 60–110 |
| CIDER | | | | | |
| Sweet | 1 glass (8 oz.) | 240 | 25 | trace | 100 |
| Hard (fermented) | 1 wine glass (3½ oz.) | 100 | 1 | 5 | 40 |

*Examples of dry wine include bordeaux, claret, graves, dry sauterne, burgundy, chablis, dry champagne, Rhine wine, and moselle.

• Don't get stressed out if your hostess serves food cooked with wine. The carbohydrate addition is negligble and most of the alcohol is lost in the cooking. If you take Diabinese and you suffer from the "Antabuse effect," however, then you must be more careful. Ask questions before you eat.

## RATING THE POPULAR DIETS

Now for a brief discussion of some of the diets that are popular today. Are they good for you?

• *Vegetarian* diets have become popular in America, among diabetics as well as the rest of the population. Type 1 diabetics who become vegetarians may need less insulin. Type 2s may lose weight on these diets and so improve their blood-glucose control. Will they work for you? They can, *if* you consult a dietitian for advice before you begin and are vigilant about your blood-sugar levels. You must eat a diet balanced in carbohydrates, fats, and proteins and this is not a simple matter if you don't eat meat or fish.

It is recommended that you do not follow a strict vegetarian diet, eliminating all animal foods and eating only plants. To get the needed supply of protein, strict vegetarians consume combinations of vegetables and grains that will far exceed the levels of carbohydrate that are safe for you. Besides, this diet puts you in danger of deficiencies of important vitamins and minerals.

If your diet allows fish, eggs, and/or dairy products, being a vegetarian is not quite as tricky, though tricky it remains. The protein plant foods used to supplement fish and dairy foods are very high in carbohydrate. For example, it takes only ⅛ cup of cooked lentil, mung, pinto, red beans, or chick peas, or ¼ cup of soy beans, to equal about 15 grams of carbohydrate.

You must take care not to consume too many grams of carbohydrate at any one time, especially not too many of the quickly absorbed variety. The usual large amounts of carbohydrate in a vegetarian diet can easily cause problems with your blood-sugar level, though the increased fiber may give you a little more leeway.

• *The popular high-protein diets:* We would all like to lose weight quickly when we are too heavy, not just a pound or two a week as our doctors and the more sensible weight-loss diets suggest. Are quick diets safe for you?

They may be safe for mild diabetics if you stay on them for only two weeks at the outside, if your health is good, if you are under medical supervision, and if you have your own doctor's approval.

The Atkins diet and other quickies that feature high protein and low carbohydrate can be dangerous, though if you are on oral agents or diet alone you can probably get away with them for a short time. Some people will even lose their dependency on oral agents while they are on one of these diets. But the high-protein diets are not safe for more severe diabetics because they are designed to burn fat and produce a state of acidosis, just what you must avoid. Remember, acidosis inhibits the action of insulin and can put you right in the hospital.

• *Low-salt diets:* If your doctor has told you to lower your salt intake, then you must avoid every food high in salt even if it is otherwise permissible. Dry cereals, for example, tend to be high in salt as are processed meats, canned vegetables, and soups. Look for the low-salt or salt-free varieties.

• *Low-potassium diets:* Certain fruits, such as figs, pineapples, apples, raisins, and prunes, that are recommended for kidney disease are not recommended for you because their sugar is too readily absorbed. Stay with the fruits that have low potassium *and* are permissible for you, such as cranberry juice, grapefruit, grapes, peaches, berries, tangerines, pears, plums, watermelon, nectarines.

## CARBOHYDRATE VALUES OF POPULAR FOODS

| Food | Amount | Carbohydrate Content (Grams) |
|---|---|---|
| Almonds | ½ cup, shelled | 14 |
| Apple | 1 medium, raw | 20 |
| Artichoke, boiled | 4 oz. | 11 |
| Artichoke hearts | 5–6 hearts, 3 oz. | 22 |
| Anchovies | 1 oz. | 0.1 |
| Avocado | ½ fruit | 6.4 to 10.8 |
| Bacon | 2 slices | 0.2 |
| Baked beans | ½ cup | 20–30 |
| Bamboo shoots | ½ lb., raw | 3.4 |
| Banana | 1 small | 21 |
| Bean sprouts | ½ cup, raw | 3 |
| Beans, black | 4 oz., dry | 69 |
| Beans, green or wax, fresh, boiled | ½ cup | 3.5 |
| Beans, Italian | ½ cup | 5 |
| Beans, lima, boiled | ½ cup | 17–21 |
| Beans, pinto | ½ cup, dry | 61 |
| Beans, lentil | ½ cup, dry | 58 |
| Beans, garbanzo (chick peas) | ½ cup, dry | 61 |
| Beef pie, frozen | 8 oz. | 40 |
| Beef, consommé or broth | 1 cup | 2.7 |
| Beets, cooked | ½ cup | 7.4 |
| Bread crumbs | 1 tbsp. | 4.7 |
| Buckwheat groats | 1 oz. | 21 |
| Cashew nuts | ½ cup | 20 |
| Catsup | 1 tbsp. | 4.9 |
| Cheesecake | ⅙ of 8″ cake | 38.8 |
| Chestnuts, fresh, shelled | 3 large | 10 |
| Chicken pie | 8 oz. | 50 |
| Chili sauce | 1 tbsp. | 4.6 |

| Food | Amount | Carbohydrate Content (Grams) |
|---|---|---|
| Coconut, fresh | ½ cup, grated | 3.8 |
| Coconut, dried, sweetened | ½ cup | 23 |
| Cornstarch | 1 tbsp. | 7 |
| Cracker crumbs, graham | 1 cup | 76.6 |
| Curry powder | 1 tbsp. | 4.9 |
| Dates | 5 | 40.5 |
| Eggnog | ½ cup | 17 |
| Fig, fresh | 1, small | 7.6 |
| Flour | 1 oz. | 21 |
| Frankfurter | 1 | 0.7 |
| Gefilte fish, canned | 1 piece, 4 oz. | 4.2 |
| Lasagne, canned | 8 oz. | 29.7 |
| frozen with meat sauce | 7½ oz. | 43 |
| Lemon juice, fresh | 1 lemon | 4 |
| Mango, fresh | 1 medium | 33.6 |
| Matzoh meal | 1 cup | 94 |
| Mayonnaise | 1 tbsp. | 0.2 |
| Milk, condensed, sweetened | 1 cup | 166 |
| Milk, evaporated | 1 cup | 24 |
| Milk, whole, skim, or buttermilk | 1 cup | 12 |
| Oil | | 0 |
| Onion, raw, chopped | ½ cup | 7.5 |
| Papaya | 4 oz. | 11.3 |
| Peanuts | ½ cup, shelled | 13 |
| Peanut butter | 1 tbsp. | 2–4 |
| Pecans | ½ cup, shelled | 7.9 |
| Pimiento, canned | 4 oz. | 6.6 |
| Pizza, home baked, with cheese | 4 oz. | 32 |

| Food | Amount | Carbohydrate Content (Grams) |
|------|--------|------------------------------|
| Popcorn, plain | 1 cup | 10.7 |
| Potato chips | 1 oz. | 14 |
| Raisins, whole | ½ cup | 55.7 |
| Ravioli, canned, beef | 1 cup | 28.3 |
| Relish, hot-dog | 1 tbsp. | 5 |
| Sardines, canned in oil | 3 oz. | 0 |
| Sesame seeds, dry, whole | 1 oz. | 6.1 |
| Soybean curd | 4 oz. | 2.7 |
| Soy milk | 8 oz. | 4.3 |
| Succotash, frozen | ½ cup | 19 |
| Sugar | 1 tbsp. | 12.1 |
| Sunflower seeds, hulled | 1 oz. | 5.6 |
| Sweet potato, peeled | 1 medium | 38 |
| Tomato, fresh | 1 medium | 7 |
| Tomato juice | ½ cup | 5.2 |
| Tomato paste | 6 oz. | 31 |
| Tomato purée | 1 cup | 22 |
| Tomato sauce | 1 cup | 20 |
| Vegetable juice cocktail, canned | 4 oz. | 4.1 |
| Vegetables, mixed, frozen | ½ cup | 12 |

# EXERCISE: ESSENTIAL FOR DIABETICS

Better to hunt in Fields, for Health unbought,
than fee the doctor for a nauseous Draught.
The Wise, for Cure, on exercise depend;
God never made his Work, for Man to mend.

—JOHN DRYDEN

Y ou have to have buried yourself up to your eyebrows and worn earmuffs not to know that exercise is good for you. Everyone in America today seems to be involved in fitness programs of one variety or another, from yoga to running, and that includes plenty of diabetics. We all know now that regular vigorous exercise strengthens the cardiovascular system, lowers "bad" LDL cholesterol levels in the blood while raising the "good" HDL fats, tones your muscles, improves your circulation, lowers your blood pressure and heart rate, promotes a sense of well-being, and burns off excess weight.

That is quite a list of benefits, but exercise is especially good medicine for most diabetics who, because they have a special tendency toward overweight, poor circulation, high cholesterol and tryglycerides, elevated blood pressure, blood clots and accelerated arteriosclerosis, need all the help they can get.

But exercise does even more for you. It can actually help keep your diabetes under control and lower your insulin requirements. In fact, in an eleven-year study of 652 type 2 diabetics, UCLA researchers found that regular exercise and a stringent diet were enough in many cases to keep blood sugar in check without medication. In other words, enough to lower their glucose level to the nondiabetic range so they did not require oral medication or insulin injections.

Exercise has been called "invisible insulin," and that's just what it is. The more exercise you get, if you are in good health, the less insulin you are likely to require and the more stable your diabetes will probably be. Besides, you can eat more when you exercise more. As one of the early diabetologists once said, "through the sweat of your brow you can earn your bread."

Exercise lowers the level of glucose circulating in your bloodstream. Muscles use glucose as their fuel, first consuming whatever is in the blood, then calling on the liver to deliver more from its stores of glycogen, using it faster than it can be produced. Unless this is carried to an extreme, it is obviously a fine feature for a diabetic who has the chronic problem of glucose disposal. There is evidence, too, that this improved glucose tolerance tends to last for a number of hours after exercise, sometimes even through the next day. A young person requires only about 15 or 20 minutes of jogging a day, and an older person only 10 minutes of brisk walking two or three times a day to bring sugar levels down significantly.

Be sure, however, to check your blood-glucose level before you start doing heavy physical exercise. If your sugar level is high, over 250 or 270 mgs percent before you begin, it may rise even higher rather than decrease.

With exercise, insulin is also more readily taken up by the body's cells because of an increase in both insulin sensitivity and the actual number of receptors on target cells in muscle, fat, and liver tissue. A study at Yale University Medical Center demonstrated a 30 percent rise in insulin sensitivity and a 50 percent increase in the number of insulin cell receptors among a group of subjects after a six-week program of daily physical training.

Another study, conducted in Denmark, shows a similar increase in glucose tolerance and insulin intake among diabetics who exercised every morning.

If you are ready for another documented reason to get exercise, here it is: regular physical activity can reduce your risk of developing the diabetic eye changes called retinopathy and other vascular diabetic complications. Many diabetics have an abnormal tendency toward "sticky" blood platelets, platelets that clump together and form clots. Research at the University of California Medical Center in San Francisco found that, for both type 1 diabetics and normal individuals, there is a significant drop in this stickiness with exercise, an effect that tends to last many hours.

Other researchers who measured the biochemical response to a blockage of veins in healthy adults before and after they participated in a ten-week conditioning program confirmed that regular vigorous exercise improves the ability to dissolve blood clots.

Caution: If you already have retinopathy, this may be another story and vigorous exercise may not be wise. Be especially cautious if you lift weights—never lift them above eye level (see Chapter 11).

## A BALANCING ACT

Diabetes control is always a balancing act between intake (food), which must contain enough glucose to fuel the body, and outgo (bodily functions and exercise, perhaps aided by insulin or oral agents). Your doctor always tries to determine how active you are before deciding on the amount of medication you must take. If you don't exercise, you'll need less food and/or more medication than someone in exactly the same medical situation who exercises.

To make this balancing act work (and to keep life simple), it is always best to get approximately the same amount of exercise every day. That way you will know just how much medication you need to take, as well as what to eat. Otherwise, you must make constant adjustments.

But if you are a working person, you probably sit at a desk most of the week and do your exercise on weekends, or maybe you only get out to run or bike or walk every few days. In this case, you have to plan ahead, one day at a time. Some people have two different diets, one for sedentary days, another for active days. If they take insulin, they sometimes inject different amounts as well. Unless you are spilling a lot of sugar (never a good idea), you always run the risk if you take insulin of an insulin reaction when you exercise. This is the number one concern of diabetic athletes.

If you don't take insulin, life is obviously a whole lot easier. First, you don't have to be so careful about eating on time. Second, after you have burned up your sugar you will have less extraneous insulin in your bloodstream to cause a reaction. Even if you take oral medication, reactions won't be a problem for you. Oral medication is not oral insulin, and it is extremely rare for people who don't take insulin to have insulin shock unless they are very ill and debilitated, or haven't eaten at all for a long period of time.

## AVOIDING REACTIONS

Let's face it, if you take insulin and your diabetes is in good control—which should always be your goal—you may have to experience an occasional insulin reaction. This is preferable to constant high blood sugar, which will eventually take its toll on your body (see Chapter 11). Ideally, you are taking enough insulin to cover your food and your activities and keep your sugar level normal. When you exercise more than usual, you burn off extra glucose and may become hypoglycemic unless you take precautionary measures.

On a day when you are going to exercise heavily, you must plan ahead. Either take less insulin or eat more food, or both. This is something you must work out with your own doctor, because everyone's requirements are different; usually an insulin reduction of about 20 percent works out satisfactorily if it is combined with an increase in protein and carbohydrate. Don't ever try to make adjustments without your doctor's advice as well as constant blood tests to be sure you are not going from one blood-sugar extreme to the other.

Let's take an example. You plan to run this morning. You test your blood and it is normal or low.

If you take Regular and Intermediate-acting insulin in combination, reduce your Regular dose by 20 percent (if your doctor agrees), or if it is a small dose omit the Regular insulin and at breakfast eat 10 to 20 *extra* grams of carbohydrate *plus* some protein that will slowly convert to carbohydrate in a few hours.

If you take only Intermediate insulin, cut back a few units and increase your food.

When you decide to do your heavy physical activity in the afternoon, remember that Intermediate-acting insulin peaks around 3 P.M. You probably should reduce your Intermediate dose that morning by 20 percent or by whatever amount you and your doctor have decided works best for you.

## SOME ALTERNATIVE ARRANGEMENTS

• For some people a more workable plan is to take the usual dose of insulin, then to add more food to make up the difference, especially when activities aren't predictable in advance.

• For overweight diabetics, lowering the insulin intake is probably better than adding calories. This way, you can lose weight at the same time.

• Now, suppose you plan to exercise today and when you test your blood you see an elevated blood-sugar level. If it isn't excessively high, you can use the exercise to help your insulin bring down the sugar. Take your normal dose and eat a little less carbohydrate at the meal before you start off.

• If, on the other hand, you are going to be exercising *really* rigorously, the recommendation is to take your full complement of food and assume the exercise itself will act like extra insulin.

• Exception: if you wake up with diabetic acidosis, or near-acidosis, exercise will aggravate your situation. If your sugar level is up to around 250 or 270 mgs, call off your plans. That's easy, because you won't feel like going through with them anyway.

## SNACKING FOR SAFETY

A carbohydrate or protein-and-carbohydrate snack about a half hour before the run or the game is recommended if your blood sugar is normal or low. Again, you must work this out with your doctor or by trial and error.

Sometimes planning ahead isn't enough. Perhaps you'll need some quick-acting carbohydrate *during* your exercise. If the tennis match goes into the fourth or fifth set and you still haven't won, your breakfast or lunch plus a snack may not be enough to get you through. Stop for a few seconds, take out some of your emergency rations, which you must *always* carry with you, and have a snack to boost your blood sugar. If you're playing golf, plan to snack at the ninth hole. Don't wait for the eleventh or twelfth or you may be sorry.

For most people, a small amount of carbohydrate about every 20 minutes during very hard exercise is sufficient. You'll soon get a sense of how much you need, and how often. A pitcher for the old Boston Braves had it all worked out in peanuts. If he had to throw more pitches or give up more hits than he'd anticipated, he ate extra peanuts based on the number of balls thrown at the plate.

Along with carbohydrate to counteract low blood sugar, you must also replace lost fluids. Your body needs the fluid you have lost through sweating. Drink plenty of water. Avoid the commercial electrolyte glucose drinks—they are too concentrated for you and may interfere with the rate at which sugar gets into your bloodstream.

Don't wait for a warning that an insulin reaction is coming; sometimes there is none. Anticipate. If you're a newcomer to diabetes or exercise, remember you will soon be able to tell when it is time for a booster. Suppose you are playing baseball. Instead of striking out and sitting down on the bench in your usual fashion, you make a three-base hit. Now you've got to make a mad sprint around the bases. Or you're late for the 5:45 train and run a few blocks to catch it. You haven't planned on it and so you have not adjusted your food or your medication. This is the time to pull out those emergency rations from your pocket and eat them.

Just a *small* amount of food will do the job. If you need more in 15 minutes, take a little more (see Chapter 9). Many people panic and overshoot the mark, taking too much sugar to ward off a reaction. While they may have made the train or won the ball game, now they have to pay the price of very high sugar which may be harder to cope with than the other extreme.

It's best to exercise *after* a meal, though obviously you should give yourself time to do a little digesting first. After you have eaten, your blood-sugar level is on the rise. Before a meal, it may be very low. For most people who take insulin, the best time to exercise is in the morning after breakfast. But if you can only work out in midafternoon, remember that your longer-acting insulin is peaking at that moment. Besides considering lowering your morning dose, be sure to have a snack first and be on the lookout for reactions.

## CHECK IT OUT

When you are on insulin, it's essential to test your blood for an up-to-the-minute report before going out to do heavy exercise. If it tests low before you even begin, you will know you need some carbohydrate for sure.

If you'll be driving yourself home after a tennis match or an aerobic stint, check your blood before you get into the car. If you're going to drive more than a half-hour, stop for a snack. You are much more likely to get where you're going if you take precautions.

## THE IMPORTANCE OF SHAPING UP

When you first start an exercise program, don't leap right in and go at it strenuously. Work up to it slowly, after a discussion with your doctor (yes, yes, yes, talk to your doctor even about this), and if you are over forty, you need a cardiovascular assessment before you begin.

There's probably no reason you can't participate in any kind of sports or exercise like anyone else, but you must give yourself time to adjust your food and medication requirements and to get your body in condition. Sudden strenuous exercise is dangerous for anyone, especially for diabetics.

For most people, aerobic exercise, the kind that makes your heart and lungs work harder, is recommended at least three times a week for at least thirty minutes a day. To burn calories and increase muscle tone, your desired heart rate should be 85 percent of 220 minus your age. Avoid high-impact activities if you have eye or nerve damage, but walking, swimming, and biking are good choices for almost everyone.

## EXERCISE MAY NOT BE FOR YOU

Though everyone needs a certain amount of physical activity to burn calories and sugar, vigorous exercise is not recommended for some diabetics. That's why it is always imperative to consult your physician before you set out to be an athlete. If your diabetes is in poor control, you may do yourself more harm than good. Studies have shown that, rather than lowering blood glucose as in well-controlled people, prolonged strenuous exercise may *raise* your sugar level as well as increase the production of ketones. So it may actually aggravate your diabetes.

Exercise may also be contraindicated for you if you have certain diabetic complications. Obviously, foot or leg problems may be one of these (again this is individual—sometimes exercise is very helpful in promoting circulation in these areas). Others may include, for example, retinopathy, because rising blood pressure during exercise may cause hemorrhaging; kidney disease because exercise increases albumin excretion; heart disease because of the danger of overexerting (exercise may be just what you need, however, but only under medical supervision and with a program tailor-made for you).

## CHOOSING THE RIGHT INJECTION SITE

One simple way to help avoid hypoglycemia (insulin reaction) when you exercise is to remember that *where* you inject yourself can make all the difference. If you will be using your legs—running, biking—then you should not inject your insulin in a leg that day because it will be absorbed more rapidly, perhaps precipitating a reaction. If you will be using your right arm, choose your left for your injection today. Remember, too, that injections in the arms or abdomen—if these are not your customary sites—can also absorb much more quickly than those in the legs. So you may have to reduce your dose by a few units, unless your sugar is high, if you make a switch to these new areas.

As a general rule, however, it is always best to take your shots in one area, such as the abdomen, because the results will tend to be more uniform.

## BEWARE THE "MONDAY SYNDROME"

After some really heavy exercise, your insulin requirements may remain at a lower level the following day while your muscles replenish their supplies of glucose and your liver stocks up on glycogen again. You may need to eat more (or take less insulin) to compensate for this. Again, individual judgment is required here because it is true for some diabetics and not others.

## KEEP A WEATHER WATCH

Your food and insulin needs may also be affected by heat or cold, either of which can make you burn more energy and therefore become more susceptible to a reaction.

## GET A BUDDY

It is never smart to be alone when you are doing the kind of exercise that may produce a reaction. Activities such as skiing, running, swimming, or sailing can be dangerous if no one is around when you need help. Anyway, they are more fun when you have company, so find yourself a fellow athlete. Let that person know you have diabetes and explain what to do if you have a reaction (see Chapter 9).

## CHECK OUT YOUR WARDROBE

The right gear is important for any sport or exercise, but when you are a diabetic you especially want to avoid certain things—overheating, sore feet, sunburn. Wear the proper shoes for your sport, making sure they fit well, do not rub, and are well cushioned. Under them, wear absorbent heavy-duty socks that fit smoothly. No lumps. No holes. Check your feet every night for blisters or other injuries. Don't exercise with feet that look like trouble. Watch all of this because diabetics are particularly susceptible to potentially serious circulatory problems (see Chapter 11). Wear layers of clothes so you can shed some if you need to.

## DANGER: FROSTBITE

When participating in winter sports, remember to take special care of your hands and feet. If you have poor circulation, this can be vitally important—frostbite is not what you need. Wear a warm hat, lined gloves, wool socks, and warm boots. Go inside frequently and check your fingers and toes (as well as your face and ears) to be sure there is no change in color or sensation. Frostbite means a quick trip to the doctor. Don't try to deal with it yourself. If a doctor isn't immediately available, however, immerse the frostbitten area in lukewarm (never hot) water or cover it with a clean cloth or blanket until you see the doctor.

## REMEMBER YOUR SUPPLIES

Be sure whatever you are wearing has pockets, because you will need a place to stash concentrated quick-acting sugar, glucose gel or tablets, or a small carbohydrate snack, along with your identification card. If you have no pockets, stash a few glucose tablets in your socks just above your ankle. That's where surgeons like to keep their wallets in the operating room. Some people like to wear a belt designed to hold sugar or candy, the card, and even a small plastic bottle for a drink. Others hang a plastic pouch of supplies on their belts. Of course, if you are going to be in one place, such as a tennis court, you can carry your goodies in a separate bag.

## NO ALCOHOLIC CELEBRATIONS

Many people feel that a nip of wine, a shot of whiskey, or a few beers on the ski slopes or at the finish of a tough bout on the playing field is only what they deserve. But athletics and alcohol don't mix, especially for diabetics. Exercise lowers your blood sugar. At the same time, alcohol inhibits the release of glucose from the liver in response to that low blood sugar, and so it may have quite a different effect than you expect. Right now, you need the glucose from your liver to fuel your brain and replenish your supply. If you drink, you may have an insulin reaction then and there. Give up the nip for a little protein or carbohydrate.

## HOW MUCH IS ENOUGH?

Here's how much exercise you should do five days a week to burn off about 2,000 calories:

| | |
|---|---|
| Swimming | 30 minutes a day |
| Aerobic exercise | 40 minutes a day |
| Tennis (singles) | 57 minutes a day |
| Running | 30 minutes a day |
| Walking (4.4 mph) | 60 minutes a day |

If you get an hour's lunch break, eat for 45 minutes and take a 15-minute brisk walk. You could lose 1,000 to 1,500 calories a month—4 to 5 pounds a year.

# 6

# TAKING ORAL AGENTS

Swallowing a couple of small pills every day is much more appealing and less complicated than giving yourself insulin injections. So if the oral hypoglycemic drugs work for you, consider yourself lucky. There is little need to worry about reactions, no concern about always eating on time, no fuss and muss with needles and syringes and measuring out insulin.

The oral hypoglycemic agents are not for every diabetic because they require that your pancreas has functioning islet cells capable of secreting insulin. Type 1 or IDDM diabetics cannot benefit from them. The typical person for whom oral agents work well is a "mild" type 2 diabetic who would probably require less than 40 units of insulin, and was diagnosed after the age of forty or fifty.

The oral agents are not oral insulin. They are not even related to insulin. Instead, they are synthetic drugs that lower your blood sugar. Some of them stimulate your pancreas to recognize that the glucose level of your blood has risen and to release the appropriate insulin in response. Others lower blood sugar by inhibiting the release of glucose from the liver or increase the effectiveness of your own or injected insulin.

The drugs most commonly used today are the sulfonylureas (Orinase, Dymelor, Tolinase, Diabinese, Diabeta, Micronase, Glucotrol, Glucotrol XL, Glynase Prestab, and Amaryl). Sulfonylureas were discovered by a French scientist who was looking for an effective antibiotic and found that a type of sulfa drug had the secondary effect of lowering blood sugar. The drugs are also thought to perform an additional function: to increase the number and efficiency of the insulin receptors on muscle and fat cells, thereby allowing insulin to enter the cells and help them metabolize sugar. Think of insulin as a key and each receptor as a door. By increasing the number of doors, assuming you have enough keys, more glucose can penetrate the cell walls.

Two other kinds of oral hypoglycemic agents for diabetics were approved by the F.D.A. in 1995. They are metformin (brand name Glucophage) and acarbose (Precose), both of which lower blood sugar without raising the insulin level. Metformin decreases the liver's capacity for producing glucose, while acarbose delays the absorption of carbohydrate in the digestive system. You'll read more about these agents later in this chapter.

Theoretically, since none of these three newer oral agents increase the amount of insulin in your bloodstream, they may be healthier for you than insulin or the sulfonylureas. It's best not to have excessive insulin circulating in your body because it can result in increased blood pressure and atherosclerosis. Besides, it stimulates your appetite, often encouraging you to eat too much.

## ARE ORAL AGENTS SAFE?

According to all current evidence, oral hypoglycemic agents do *not* increase your chances of heart attack as was once feared.

Many years ago, an extensive eight-year study called the University Group Diabetes Program linked the oral hypoglycemic agents with an increased risk of death from heart disease. The study's conclusions caused many doctors to stop prescribing the pills and replace them with insulin injections if their patients' diabetes could not be controlled with diet.

These claims have now been denied by both the American Diabetic Association and the American Medical Association. Doctors who have been prescribing the oral hypoglycemics for over thirty years have found no increase in heart disease among their patients. Nor have other studies found any differences in the incidence of heart attacks.

As a result, all diabetologists today recommend the oral hypoglycemics for appropriate patients, because these drugs present far fewer problems than insulin injections do. If you are a diabetic who cannot control your diabetes with diet alone, and can achieve a normal blood-sugar level without having to take a shot every day and without having to be concerned with insulin reactions and rigid eating schedules, it definitely makes good sense to choose the pills.

## ORAL AGENTS: THE SULFONYLUREAS

There are many varieties of sulfonylureas available in the United States today. From the weakest to the strongest, they are:

*Orinase,* the first successful sulfonylurea compound on the American market, is rarely used today. The least powerful of the drugs, it is sold in 500 mg tablets. You may require only one tablet, or up to six a day in divided doses.

*Dymelor,* slightly stronger and also rarely prescribed, has a secondary effect of lowering the level of uric acid, which is high in many diabetics and could lead to kidney stones. Available in 250 and 500 mg tablets, it is given in single or divided doses up to 1,500 mgs a day.

*Tolinase,* available in 100, 250, and 500 mg tablets, is also prescribed up to 1,000 mgs a day. An advantage of this drug is its diuretic effect. Some diabetics tend to retain fluid and so this form of oral agent may be best for them. A weak-acting drug, it can provide a small boost for mild diabetics who don't need stronger agents.

*Diabinese,* the strongest of the four original oral agents, is still prescribed but not as often as the newer agents available today. It is made in 100 and 250 mg tablets and since the drug remains in the body for about 36 hours, the dose is never split but always taken at one time—before breakfast. Diabinese produces an "Antabuse effect" in some people when they consume alcohol. If this happens in your case, you will quickly develop a beet-red facial flush, a choking sensation, and perhaps a headache. This can happen even when you eat food that has been cooked in wine or liquor so you must always inquire about dishes served away from home before taking a bite. While this is a nuisance, there may be reason to consider yourself fortunate if you suffer from the Antabuse effect. Recent research shows that the diabetic who has such reactions runs a lesser risk of succumbing to retinopathy and other major cardiovascular diseases.

*Diabeta, Micronase, Glynase Prestab* (all glyburides), *Glucotrol, Glucotrol XL* (glipizides), and the newer sulfonylureas such as *Amaryl,* are the strongest and most effective oral agents today. They are all mildly diuretic. The glyburides are thought to work by decreasing the sugar released from the liver, especially fasting sugar in the morning, while the glipizides stimulate insulin production after you eat. Glynase Prestab, a pill within a pill, releases the glyburide uniformly throughout the day.

*Amaryl* (glimepiride) is a sulfonylurea too, but uses different pathways to increase the efficiency of the body's available insulin. This drug also helps prevent arteriosclerosis ("hardening of the arteries").

Diabeta and Micronase come in 1.25, 2.5, and 5 mg tablets and are prescribed up to 20 mgs a day, taken in one dose before breakfast. Glucotrol is available in 5 and 10 mg (normal and long-lasting) tablets. The UKPDS study showed no difference in complications between insulin and oral agents. Lowering blood pressure also reduced complications.

## THE NONSULFONYLUREA ORAL AGENTS

*Glucophage:* A newer oral agent for treating type 2 diabetes has become very popular today and for good reason—it has improved the lives of many mild diabetics and has several advantages over the sulfonylureas. This is metformin (sold under the brand name Glucophage), available in Europe and Canada for over 30 years before its approval in the United States in 1995. This drug is one of the biguanides, a class of drugs derived from a plant called goat's rue or French lilac and used in the Middle Ages for medicinal purposes. This author was among the first to discover that it lowers cholesterol, triglycerides, and weight as well as blood sugar.

Unlike the sulfonylureas, metformin does not work by stimulating insulin secretion. Instead it suppresses the liver's production of glucose by up to 75 percent, reducing levels circulating in the bloodstream. At the same time, it increases your own insulin's ability to metabolize sugar up to 29 percent. In other words, it is a glucose-disposal drug. When used alone, it almost never causes hypoglycemia or low blood sugar although it may when combined, as it frequently is, with a sulfonylurea or insulin. It reduces LDL and triglyceride levels and modestly increases HDL, just what the doctor ordered. Because it controls blood sugar by decreasing the amount of insulin in the bloodstream, it may decrease the risk of arteriosclerosis. Besides, it reduces blood pressure in hypertensive and nonhypertensive diabetics. Best of all, unlike sulfonylureas or insulin, it does not cause weight gain.

Taken with meals in doses of 500 to 2,500 mgs spaced out over a day, Glucophage sometimes produces side effects—nausea, diarrhea, metallic taste—which usually dissipate within a couple of weeks. If they don't, this drug is not for you. Nor is it for you if you have liver or kidney disease, metabolic acidosis, or congestive heart failure; and it is not recommended for alcoholics, children, or pregnant women. If you have an IVP (intravenous pyelogram) or a CT scan with contrast, you must stop taking it for two days after the procedure. According to the United Kingdom Prospective Diabetes Study in 1998, this was the only diabetic drug shown to reduce the incidence of fatal heart attacks when used alone. A Glucophage XR, to be taken with the biggest meal once a day, supposedly gives less gastrointestinal side effects.

*Precose:* Another recently approved oral agent is acarbose (brand name Precose), a drug that is usually used in combination with insulin or sulfonylurea agents and probably is most appropriate for diabetics who aren't quite making it with the other medications. Acarbose or Precose works by delaying the digestion of carbohydrates in the small intestine, thus preventing a surge in blood glucose after meals and giving the pancreas more time to pump out enough insulin. Not as potent as metformin or the sulfonylureas, it is taken with the first bite of the meal and may be used alone or in combination with other oral agents or insulin. Precose has a few gastrointestinal side effects, most noticeably flatulence and diarrhea, which usually diminish over time. It should always be taken with a meal. It is not recommended for those with kidney disease or intestinal problems. If you weigh less than 130 pounds, don't take a dose greater than 150 mgs a day. With the new drug Glyset (miglitol), you may take the standard dose regardless of your weight.

*Glitazones:* Called insulin sensitizers, glitazones were designed to help poorly controlled type 2 diabetics make better use of the insulin made naturally in their own bodies or taken through injections. They lower insulin resistance by increasing the absorption of sugar by fat tissue and muscle and, in high doses, reduce the amount of sugar released by the liver into the bloodstream. Rezulin (troglitazone), the first drug in this class, was taken off the market due to possible liver damage. Actos (pioglitazone) and Avandia (rosiglitazone) can cause liver toxicity too, and so must be monitored regularly by liver blood tests. Occasionally they also cause edema and anemia and should not be used if you have severe heart disease. They may prevent cardiac damage by influencing clotting.

*Nonsulfonylureas* are similar to sulfonylureas but do not contain sulfa. These include Prandin (repaglinide) and Starlix (nateglinide), both of which work more quickly than sulfa drugs but do not last as long, so there is less chance of hypoglycemia.

ORAL HYPOGLYCEMIC AGENTS

| Trade name | Generic name | Size | Usual Daily Dosage |
|---|---|---|---|
| Orinase | Tolbutamide | 500 mg | 500 to 3,000 mg |
| Dymelor | Acetohexamide | 250 mg and 500 mg | 250 to 1,500 mg |
| Tolinase | Tolazamide | 100 mg, 250 mg, and 500 mg | 100 to 1,000 mg |
| Diabinese | Chlorpropamide | 100 mg and 250 mg | 100 to 500 mg |
| Diabeta | Glyburide | 1.25 mg, 2.5 mg, and 5 mg | 1.25 to 10 mg |
| Micronase | Glyburide | 1.25 mg, 2.5 mg, and 5 mg | 1.25 to 10 mg |
| Glucotrol | Glipizide | 5 mg and 10 mg | 5 to 10 mg |
| Glucotrol XL | Glipizide | 5 mg and 10 mg | 5 to 10 mg |
| Glynase Prestab | Glyburide | 1.5 mg, 3 mg, and 6 mg | 1.5 to 12 mg |
| Amaryl | Glimepiride | 1 mg, 2 mg, and 4 mg | 4 mg |
| Glucophage | Metformin | 500 mg and 850 mg | 500 to 2,500 mg |
| Precose | Acarbose | 50 mg and 100 mg | 150 to 300 mg |
| Glyset | Miglitol | 25 mg, 50 mg, and 100 mg | 25 to 300 mg |
| Prandin | Repaglinide | 0.5 mg, 1 mg, and 2 mg before each feeding | 0.5 to 8 mg |
| Starlix | Nateglinide | 120 mg before each feeding (not to be used with sulfonylureas) | 120 mg to 360 mg |
| Avandia | Rosiglitazone | 4 mg, 8 mg | 8 mg |
| Actos | Pioglitazone | 15 mg, 30 mg, and 45 mg | 15 to 45 mg |

Of all the oral agents listed above, your doctor will be able to advise you on which ones are suitable for you. Most doctors are employing more than one drug for each patient.

## DIET IS STILL IMPORTANT

Just because you are taking oral agents instead of insulin does not mean that you are home free. You still cannot eat whatever you like. Hot fudge sundaes are still not an option, at least not very often, nor is too much food of any kind. For any diabetic, diet is the most important part of the therapy. The pills will not transform you into a normal person with a normal pancreas that turns out as much insulin as you need to respond to an overload of sugar.

If you eat too much, you—just like an insulin-dependent diabetic—may end up in the hospital in a coma. Not only that, but if your diabetes is consistently out of control, even to a degree that isn't obvious to you, you are greatly increasing your risk of developing diabetic complications in the future. Just like an insulin-dependent person, you are a real diabetic. However, if you maintain your proper weight, eat sensibly, and get enough exercise, it is possible you may no longer need the oral agents and will not be considered diabetic but merely someone with a tendency toward the disease.

Extra pills are not like extra insulin. Many people think, if they overdose on food, they can compensate by taking extra pills. They cannot. They will simply go out of control and have high blood sugar, which is just as harmful to them as to any other diabetic. When your fixed maximum effect has been reached, additional pills will do no good.

## TALLY YOUR TESTS

You must also test your blood regularly. If you are well controlled, you should make tests twice a day—before breakfast and before bed or before supper. If you are not, test three or four times a day until your sugar is down. Keep a record of the results and take this to your doctor. Together you can decide how to change your diet and/or your activities so you may not have to switch to insulin.

Illnesses, excessive sugar in your diet, less exercise, more stress, etc., can cause you to spill sugar and perhaps acetone. If your sugar is high, always test for acetone in the urine. If acetone is present, confer with your doctor. A temporary supplement of insulin may be what you need. Going over to insulin during an illness or pregnancy does not make you insulin-dependent. When you no longer need the shots, you can probably return to your former regime.

## WHEN YOU ARE SICK

Whenever you have an infection, especially when it is accompanied by a fever, your insulin requirements will rise. That's because not only does your liver release extra glucose as part of the body's defenses against attack but more glucose is formed from protein when you are under stress. Now you may not get enough insulin response from your pill-primed pancreas to handle this increased sugar. If your tests show prolonged high sugars, something must be done to avoid acidosis.

Your doctor will probably suggest, if you normally take only a small amount of oral medication, that you are vigilant about your diet and perhaps raise your dosage to increase the pills' efficiency. When you are already taking your maximum effective dose, however, taking more is not the answer. You have reached your limit of insulin production.

If your blood sugar does not return to normal, you'll need to turn to insulin temporarily, alone or as a supplement. Unless you are an old hand at this, do nothing on your own. Let your doctor make the decisions. Probably 5 to 10 units of Regular insulin every two hours will turn the tide.

That is why you must know how to give yourself injections and keep a bottle of Regular insulin stored in your refrigerator (replace it when it becomes outdated). Your doctor will tell you how often to take it.

Temporary insulin injections will also be needed by most diabetics on oral agents when they have major surgery. The reason is the same—increased need for insulin during stress. Sometimes, too, you may need insulin injections when you are sick and can't tolerate anything—including your oral agents—by mouth.

## POSSIBLE SIDE EFFECTS OF THE ORAL AGENTS

Once in a while, a diabetic reacts unfavorably to the oral hypoglycemic agents. The possible side effects include nausea and other gastrointestinal problems, fever, skin rashes, itching. If these symptoms do not diminish and then disappear at your lowest possible dosage, the only solution is to try other oral agents, switch over to insulin, or watch your diet more strictly.

## ARE REACTIONS A CONCERN?

Hypoglycemic reactions are an *extremely* rare occurrence when you take oral agents because your pancreas is sensitized to respond only to the glucose content of your bloodstream. The insulin does not pour out as soon as you swallow your pills, as it does from an injection, but waits until it is required.

But reactions *are* possible. Too high a dosage, unexpected and very heavy exercise, consistent insufficiency of food (especially among the elderly, who may not have a sufficient store of glycogen), can all trigger a hypoglycemic reaction. Usually the reaction is mild and easily reversible because your blood sugar does not drop as far or as fast as it would if you were taking insulin. It may make you feel weak, trembly, faint, or headachy.

Very severe reactions can occur, however, and can be much worse than reactions from insulin because they may be sudden, prolonged—perhaps lasting for days—and life-threatening. Although they are sometimes the result of overlapping effects of long-acting oral agents, they are more likely to happen when a diabetic continues to take the pills but does not eat or has a gastrointestinal upset.

Often people think that, because their diabetes responds to the pills and does not require insulin shots, they can be lackadaisical about monitoring their blood sugar. However, they must pay attention, make sure to eat enough food to cover the medication, and check their blood sugar at least twice a day.

Sometimes reactions happen for other reasons too. Liver or kidney disease, for example, can affect the behavior of the oral agents. And so can the interaction of other drugs that are detoxified in the liver. These include:

Coumadin (an anticoagulant)
Butazolidine (an anti-inflammatory)
Sulfonamides (antibiotics)
Benemid (for gout)
Dilantin (for epilepsy)
Mood amelioratiors such as MAO inhibitors

The treatment for hypoglycemia is always the same—eat some quickly absorbed carbohydrate, along with some protein. Because the hypoglycemia may not be reversed quickly if it is due to overlapping doses of oral agents or disease, your blood sugar should be closely monitored until you're back to normal.

Be *sure* to inform any doctor who treats you that you are diabetic and take oral agents, so that this will be taken into account if other drugs are prescribed.

*Never* skip your meals, and remember to eat extra food if you are going to engage in heavy exercise.

Tell your doctor if you ever have reactions. Because reactions are so rare when you take oral agents, it is most important to know the reason for them.

## OTHER DRUG INTERACTIONS

Inderal and other beta blockers, drugs prescribed for hypertension, can block the secretion of insulin and cause the oral agent to be ineffective in some cases. Nevertheless, it may be necessary to use beta blockers in certain heart conditions, in which case you may have to adjust your dose or switch to insulin.

And the effects of most barbiturates, sedatives, and hypnotics can be seriously prolonged when you take sulfonylurea agents.

## WILL THE PILLS EVER BECOME INEFFECTIVE?

For most people, the oral agents continue to do their job indefinitely. Though it was once thought that their effect always diminished after five or ten years, it has been found that only 17 percent of pill-takers have "secondary failure" and must start taking insulin instead.

If your diabetes control seems to be worse, the most likely explanation is that you aren't paying attention to your diet or your need for exercise. Neither pills nor insulin shots will keep you from all the problems of diabetes without proper living habits. But if you are in the minority whose internal insulin production does diminish with time, a stronger or longer-acting oral agent may help reestablish your control. Not only that, but today, with so many new oral agents available, it is possible to combine these drugs so that they'll do a better job of keeping your blood sugar within normal boundaries. If this doesn't work, then you must turn to insulin.

But before switching you over to a total insulin regime, your diabetic specialist may decide to try BIDS (bedtime insulin/daytime sulfonylureas) in case that's all you need. This means that you take your usual oral agents during the day and add a little insulin at bedtime. This works very well for many people although it makes insulin reactions more likely. Keep in mind that reactions when you are on oral agents—especially when insulin is added—can be very severe, so you must be especially vigilant about your blood-sugar levels.

## IF YOU FORGET TO TAKE YOUR DOSE

It is not a good idea to omit your dose of oral agent and you should *never* stop taking it because you're feeling better, but it isn't a serious matter if you forget to take it only once in a while. That is because you do make some insulin on your own, and a brief period without the agent won't raise your blood sugar to dangerous levels. Simply take your pill when you remember it. If you have gone as long as a whole day without the medication and your blood tests show high sugar, be sure to take your pill immediately. If you are very symptomatic (excessive thirst or urination), call your doctor promptly because you may be heading for acidosis.

# 7

# GOING THE
# INSULIN ROUTE

All type 1 diabetics, and those type 2s whose blood sugar cannot be controlled by diet therapy or oral agents, must take injections of insulin to replace the insulin they no longer make on their own. This means daily injections, a prospect nobody regards with great joy. But once you accept them as essential to your health, they can be managed without turning your life upside down. Eating on time, sticking to your diet, testing your blood, adjusting your dose, being alert to low blood sugar as well as high can all become routine parts of your daily existence that need not always dominate your thoughts. If insulin therapy is new to you, this may be hard to believe, but with time and experience you can learn to go about your business despite being an insulin-dependent diabetic.

Consider a diabetic's fate before this miracle drug was discovered. Before 1922, adults who developed diabetes were lucky to live another ten years, youngsters a few months. Diet was the only known treatment and starving was the alternative to diabetic coma.

In 1921, Drs. Charles Best and Frederick Banting, using research by Dr. Moses Barron, extracted a substance from a steer's pancreas and injected it into a diabetic dog, promptly lowering the dog's blood sugar. With that success, the outlook for diabetics changed overnight. Drs. Best and Banting next gave the new extract to each other, waited 24 hours, then injected it into a twelve-year-old diabetic boy who was near death but made a dramatic recovery on a steady regime of insulin injections. In only a year, Best and Banting and other scientists developed the techniques for mass-producing the miracle hormone, literally creating life for people who previously had been doomed.

## TODAY'S INSULIN

Some insulin is still extracted from pigs and cattle, but it is very different from the liquid that filled that first syringe. Animal insulin has been made more and more pure until now most of the contaminants have been removed, making it much less likely to cause allergic reactions and perhaps some of the common diabetic complications as well.

Most insulin now on the market, however, is synthesized from bacteria or yeast cells and is biologically identical to human insulin. Genetically altered by gene-splicing techniques, it not only does an excellent job but will never be in short supply, as animal insulin once was, because it can be mass-produced as needed in bacterial factories.

The manufactured insulins are combined with other substances that modify the rate at which they are absorbed, so they may be prescribed according to individual needs. The solubility of insulin, which determines how quickly it enters the bloodstream and goes into action, is decided by three factors: the physical form (amorphous or crystalline) and, if crystalline, the size of the crystals; the amount of zinc salts added; and the nature of the buffer solution holding it.

A recently approved extra-long-acting insulin called Lantus (glargine) remains active in the body for 24 hours, so one injection a day, taken at bedtime, can replace two daily injections of other long-acting insulins. In most cases, it should be used in combination with Humalog.

## WHAT'S THE NEWS?

Insulin in its present forms must be injected to be effective because taken orally it is destroyed by the digestive enzymes before it reaches the bloodstream. However, recent work at Brown University with tiny drug-filled beads that stick to intestinal tissues and slowly erode to release the drug into the bloodstream suggests that an oral insulin may be available before very long. And an inhaled insulin, another way of eliminating the need for injections, is in the works and will probably be approved by the F.D.A. very soon.

## A CURE FOR DIABETES?

Not too far in the future, diabetes may actually be cured, making any form of exogenous insulin unnecessary, by transplanting insulin-producing pancreatic islet cells into the body where they will manufacture the hormone. Scientists are working on new methods of acquiring beta cells from human, fetal, and animal sources. The cells will be grown in the laboratory, masked to prevent rejection by the body, and screened to prevent the transmission of viral diseases.

Meanwhile, researchers at the Joslin Diabetes Center in Boston and others at Vanderbilt University are focusing on the development of a membrane device to encapsulate healthy islet cells and protect them from the recipient's immune system after transplantation. The hope is that the encapsulated cells will act like an artificial pancreas, releasing insulin in response to blood-glucose levels.

Pancreatic transplants are another way to go, with more than 5,000 such procedures having been performed from 1966 to 1994. The current rate of survival for complete kidney-pancreas transplant now exceeds 76 percent at one year and 50 percent at five years. In Edmunton, Canada, researchers have successfully transplanted islet cells to type 1 diabetics using new anti-rejection drugs.

## KINDS OF INSULIN

Many varieties and strengths of insulin are now on the market, and only your doctor can prescribe which one or combination you should take and in what amounts. Everyone's needs are different and considerable trial and error are usually required before you find your proper track.

Insulins vary in several ways: how long they take to start lowering your blood sugar; how long this lowering ability lasts; when they "peak" or provide their maximum effect; and their strength.

### Fast-acting

*Regular* is clear insulin that takes effect very quickly, in less than an hour, peaks in 2 to 3 hours, and lasts a couple of hours longer than that in the bloodstream. In an emergency, Regular insulin can be given intravenously for even faster action.

Fast-acting insulins are rarely used alone on a daily basis, unless you are on a multiple-injection plan which means you inject yourself several times a day with small amounts of insulin in response to your blood-sugar level. These insulins are usually combined with intermediate forms for daily use, or used only when you need insulin in a hurry.

Regular insulin is taken before meals or large snacks to counteract the increase in blood glucose as food is absorbed. However, if you find when you test your blood sugar in the morning that it is below 70 mgs, take your insulin after the meal or perhaps take a smaller dose. Consult your doctor about this.

The fastest insulin today is Humalog (insulin lispro), which was approved by the F.D.A. in 1996 and was the first new insulin to come along in fourteen years. This new "designer" insulin gets into the bloodstream even faster than Regular insulin, mimicking more closely the normal body's production of insulin after eating. It works so quickly, peaking within an hour, that it can be injected within 15 minutes of a meal. This gives you more flexibility in your eating schedule, even one that changes day to day, because you can take it and promptly sit down and eat. That's a big advantage when you're eating at a restaurant or at a dinner party on other people's timetables. Its disadvantage is that it doesn't last as long as Regular insulin, so your dosage of long-acting 24-hour insulin may have to be increased to cover the lag time. It is not recommended for women who are pregnant or children under the age of ten. And, once opened, it should be discarded after 28 days.

By the way, under development at this writing is a long-acting Humalog as well as combinations of both the Regular and long-acting forms in a single bottle.

## Intermediate-acting

*NPH* and *Lente* are cloudy insulins that are in the intermediate group and are the most frequently prescribed of all. They last about 24 hours, start to work about 1 to 1½ hours after injection, and peak in 8 to 12 hours. This means they have a small amount of action before lunch and have their major effect in midafternoon.

The intermediates are prescribed by most diabetologists today because they cover you with insulin 24 hours a day, including your three meals and the glucose released from your liver during the night.

## Long-acting

*Ultralente* does not start working effectively for 4 to 8 hours, peaks 14 to 20 hours after the injection, and lasts 24 to 36 hours in the bloodstream. It is usually taken at bedtime to provide coverage all night and part of the next day.

Five insulins require prescriptions—U-500, Humalog, Humalog Mix 75/25, Novalog, and Lantus—with the others available over the counter.

The guide given here to the insulins currently on the market includes their *average* time curves, which are not necessarily accurate for you. Every diabetic is different and when an insulin, for example, lasts on average for 24 hours, you must understand that, for you, it may last 14 hours or 26 hours. That's why your instructions for insulin must take your lifestyle into consideration. Instructions must be carefully individualized and frequently reassessed by your physician.

Under investigation at the moment are many new forms of insulin that promise to be on the market before long. These include combination insulins and insulins that will provide an even distribution of the hormone throughout the day.

GUIDE TO INSULINS

| Name | Type | Onset | Peak Action | Duration |
|------|------|-------|-------------|----------|
| Humulin R | Regular | ½ hour | 2½–5 hours | 8 hours |
| Novolin R | Regular | ½ hour | 2½–5 hours | 8 hours |
| Humalog | Regular | 15 minutes | ½–1½ hours | 3–4 hours |
| Novolog | Regular | 10–20 minutes | 1–3 hours | 3–5 hours |
| Humulin N | NPH | 1½ hours | 4–12 hours | 24 hours |
| Novolin N | NPH | 1½ hours | 4–12 hours | 24 hours |
| Humulin L | Lente | 2½ hours | 7–15 hours | 22 hours |
| Novolin L | Lente | 2½ hours | 7–15 hours | 22 hours |
| Humulin U | Ultralente | 4–8 hours | 14–20 hours | 24–36 hours |
| Lantus | Long-acting | 40 minutes | no peak | 24 hours |

## PREMIXED INSULIN

Premixed insulin—a combination of Regular and NPH or Lente in one bottle—is commonly prescribed today. Because of the Regular, the dose starts to work quickly and because of the NPH or Lente, it lasts longer. Premixed eliminates the need to make injections from multiple bottles, a boon to some people, and tends to provide decent blood-sugar control. On the other hand, it is not as precise as individually tailored dosages.

### Premixed Insulin

| | |
|------|------|
| Humulin 70/30 | 70% NPH/30% Regular |
| Novolin 70/30 | 70% NPH/30% Regular |
| Humulin 50/50 | 50% NPH/50% Regular |
| Humalog 75/25 | 75% HPS/25% Humalog |

## INSULIN STRENGTHS

Today, in the United States, insulin is almost always prescribed in U-100 strength. This means there are 100 units of insulin per cubic centimeter (cc) of fluid. Until recently, insulin was also available in strengths of U-40 and U-80, or 40 and 80 units of insulin per cc of fluid. This was confusing to many people and mistakes in dosage were frequently made when switching from one strength to another. On the recommendation of the American Diabetes Association and other medical experts, the two lower strengths have been phased out of production in this country and virtually all doctors have stopped prescribing them.

In the meantime, remember: *a unit of insulin is always the same,* no matter what strength you use. In the early days, a unit was the amount of insulin that would lower the blood sugar of a four-pound rabbit to 45 mgs percent. Today the unit is standardized all over the world. If you are in another country where you may be able to buy only U-40 or U-80, you can use it, but you must know how to translate from one strength to the other.

A unit of one strength is interchangeable with a unit of any other. It has the same potency and blood-sugar lowering effect. What differs is the amount of solution or liquid in which the insulin is held. One cc of U-40 insulin contains 40 units of insulin. One cc of U-80 contains 80 units. One cc of U-100 contains 100 units of insulin. Therefore, one unit of U-40 is larger *in volume* (because of the water content) than a unit of U-80 or U-100, but the strength of one unit is always the same.

So, *one unit is one unit,* and can be exchanged for one unit of a different strength. BUT you must use a syringe that corresponds with the strength of your insulin (for example, a U-100 syringe for U-100 insulin—both have orange caps) in order to avoid errors.

## IN AN EMERGENCY

If you *must* use a syringe that does not correspond to your insulin, then you can make the translation. For example, if you run out of U-100 insulin, and must use U-40 (only U-40 is available in some countries) with a U-100 syringe: multiply your usual *volume* (not your units) of U-100 by 2½. This will give you an equivalent U-40 dose. In other words, you need a larger *volume* (2½ times as much) of U-40 to equal the same number of units of U-100 because it is less concentrated.

| | |
|---|---|
| 10 units on U-100 syringe | = 4 units of U-40 insulin |
| 20 | = 8 units |
| 30 | = 12 units |
| 40 | = 16 units |
| 50 | = 20 units |

## SYRINGE STRATEGY

Insulin syringes come in many sizes and shapes and it doesn't matter too much which one you use as long as you are always certain you use one that corresponds with your insulin strength. Syringes are marked U-40, U-80, and U-100, and they are color-coded to match the insulin bottles as well. U-100 syringes are available in 100-unit, 50-unit, and 30-unit sizes, the latter handy for people who take very small doses. The 100-unit syringe holds 100 units of insulin in 1 cc of liquid. Each line indicates 2 units of insulin. A 50-unit syringe holds 50 units of insulin in 0.5 cc of liquid and *each line marks only 1 unit.* A 30-unit size holds 30 units of insulin in 0.3 cc of liquid and *each line indicates 1 unit.*

Again, diabetics in this country rarely need to be concerned about matching syringes to insulin strengths because U-100 is the only strength available here.

Virtually everyone today uses disposable syringes and needles that are made of plastic. These can be used a few times (as long as the needles are sharp) without too much concern about sterility. Be sure to recap the needle after each use and don't clean it with alcohol because it will remove the slick coating that lets it slide in easily. Throw it away when it's dull or if it has touched anything but your own skin.

Today's smaller-gauge needles are slim, sharp, and specially coated to slide into the skin smoothly. The thinnest ½-inch needles—26, 27, 28, 29, or 30 gauge—cause the least discomfort and are the most popular. The thinner the needle the less discomfort it causes, so the 30-gauge is the least painful. Try them all out and decide which is best for you.

When you travel, take along a doctor's prescription for syringes and insulin plus a letter from the doctor stating that you are a diabetic. If you have problems getting supplies away from home, try a hospital emergency room.

## USING A PEN INJECTOR

If you hate to stick needles into yourself, even though they are so sharp and thin today that the prick is hardly noticeable, try a pen insulin injector. Insulin pens have become very popular, not only for this reason but also because they are so convenient, especially for those who take multiple doses a day. They are also handy for travelers. Lightweight and compact, they are small enough to fit in your pocket or handbag so you don't have to carry syringes and bottles of insulin around with you everywhere you go.

Some pen injectors are prefilled with 150 units of insulin and discarded when empty. Others use replaceable 150-unit cartridges. Five cartridges cost about the same price as one bottle of insulin. Cartridges of Regular insulin, premixed 70/30 insulin, NPH insulin, or Humalog are available. An easy-to-read dial on the pen allows you to set the number of units you want and a button triggers the disposable needle.

A few precautions: As with any insulin, the prefilled pens or cartridges must neither be frozen nor exposed to very high temperatures. Filled with Regular insulin, they need not be refrigerated if they are used up within a month; with Intermediate, within a week.

Before giving yourself a shot, shoot one or two units of insulin into the air to be sure the pen is working properly; then redial the dose. This is especially important for the Intermediate insulin. Never carry a pen with a pen needle attached unless its cover is on, because this leaves an open passageway for germs to reach the insulin.

Change the needle every time you use it because it may become clogged or contaminated. Do not wash the needle with alcohol, because you'll remove the silicone coating that makes the injection easy and painless.

Be careful not to confuse Regular insulin with NPH—remember that Regular is clear and NPH is cloudy. On the other hand, just to mix you up, Lantus (glargine) is clear, although it, too, is long-acting like NPH.

## ALLERGIC REACTIONS TO INSULIN

One problem many insulin-dependent diabetics have always had is an allergic response at the site of the injection, especially when they have just started to take insulin or when they take it only occasionally. Often it occurs six or more weeks after starting to take injections. The symptoms—redness, swelling, itchiness—are usually mild and localized and completely gone in a couple of weeks.

Allergic reactions have become almost a problem of the past because they are seldom caused by newer insulins, especially with "human insulin" that is made by gene-splicing. It may make us feel less than gods to realize that the 51 amino acids of pig insulin differ only by one amino acid from the human. The cow, on the other hand, is three amino acids, plus some hoofs and a tail, away. The human insulins, made by neither pigs nor cows but bacteria or yeast, show no difference at all from the insulin made by the human body, although occasional allergic reactions have been reported.

In the meantime, sometimes a diabetic must be desensitized to insulin by taking very small doses four or more times a day, increasing the amount very slowly until the proper dose is reached with no skin reactions. Doctors occasionally prescribe a tiny amount of antihistamine or cortisone mixed by injection into the insulin vial by the pharmacist to counteract the allergic response.


## INSULIN RESISTANCE

While these allergic diabetics are very sensitive to insulin, others are very resistant to it, requiring vast amounts before it begins to do its job of lowering sugar effectively. If you need more than 200 units a day, you are considered to be insulin-resistant. Sometimes the answer is cortisone therapy or a switch in insulins.

Insulin resistance is the result of a buildup of antibodies in response to the insulin, producing an allergy. Then other antibodies form to block the first ones. If too much of the second group is formed, it will interfere with the action of the insulin you take, making it much less effective, and you will need considerably larger doses.

The resistance may last for months or years. When it vanishes, it may do so very suddenly, so suddenly that all that insulin you are taking can give you a tremendous insulin shock. Be aware that this can happen and always be sure to carry emergency sweets, as well as a glucagon injection kit, wherever you go.


## HOW TO GIVE YOURSELF AN INJECTION

Though it seems very simple to an experienced person, injecting yourself is frightening for the beginner until you get the hang of it. Many people practice on something other than themselves—an orange, for example—until they have perfected a smooth technique. Even if you don't take insulin but control your diabetes with diet or oral agents, you must know how to inject it because a time may come—during an illness, perhaps—when you may require it temporarily.

## Getting Ready: The Materials You Need

Here's what you will need at hand:
  1. Insulin.
  2. A disposable syringe that corresponds to the strength of your insulin. You merely unwrap it, use it, and throw it away (or use it a few times before throwing it away).
  3. Alcohol (70 percent ethyl/91 percent isopropyl).
  4. Absorbent cotton or prepackaged alcohol swabs.

## Filling the Syringe with Insulin

  1. Remember to keep the needle sterile. Don't touch it with your fingers or anything else.
  2. Shake the insulin bottle gently, inverting it to make sure it is thoroughly mixed.
  3. Wipe off the rubber stopper on the top of the bottle with a piece of alcohol-soaked cotton. Do not remove the stopper from the bottle.
  4. Draw the plunger back to the mark on the syringe that corresponds with your dose of insulin. This fills the space with air.
  5. Insert the needle through the rubber stopper into the bottle. Push the plunger all the way down, pushing the air into the bottle.
  6. With the needle in the bottle, turn the bottle upside down and pull the plunger back *just beyond* the mark showing your correct dose.
  7. Slowly push the plunger back to the correct mark for your dose. This will expel the air bubbles. Don't worry about a few little bubbles. They won't hurt you. You would require much more air than that to do you in.
  8. When the syringe is filled with the correct dose, pull the needle out of the bottle. Don't let the bottle hang upright on the needle because the needle may bend.

## Mixing Two Insulins in One Syringe

Let's suppose your doctor has instructed you to take 4 Regular and 10 Lente units of insulin.

1. Draw air into the syringe up to the 10-unit line.

2. Put the needle through the center of the rubber cap of the Lente (cloudy) bottle and inject the 10 units of air into the bottle.

3. Withdraw the needle, *empty*.

4. Draw 4 units of air into the same syringe.

5. Push the needle through the rubber cap of the Regular bottle (this insulin is clear) and inject this air into the bottle.

6. Withdraw with 4 units of Regular insulin.

7. Turn Lente bottle upside down and insert the same needle into that bottle.

8. Slowly pull the plunger back to total 14 units. You now have 4 units of Regular and 10 units of Lente in your syringe.

NOTE: Humalog (Regular) must be injected immediately after mixing so it does not lose any of its strength. Regular mixed with Lente or Ultralente must also be injected immediately because, on standing, its composition can change.

## Choosing the Spot

Insulin may be injected into the *fronts* of your thighs (the most commonly chosen site); the *backs* and *sides* of your upper arms; the *front* and *sides* of your abdomen; or the *top* of your buttocks. To be sure to avoid major blood vessels or nerves, never inject into the outsides of your thighs, the lower or inner areas of the buttocks, or below the knee. Be careful to stay far away from the radial nerve that is located near your elbow. Do not inject into scar tissue, which can't absorb the insulin. Because fatty tissue provides the best locations, a really thin person will usually use the thighs or buttocks, while fatter people have more options.

The most important thing to remember is to rotate your sites. Don't inject in spots within one inch of each other in the same month. If you continually use one location, it may become hardened and scarred, or lumps of fat may appear under the skin. This is not beautiful, the needle won't go in very easily, and the insulin will not be absorbed as well as it should. This has become much less of a problem, however, since the human insulins have become widely available. Best to make a chart so you do not return to the exact same spot within a month.

The best method is to rotate around the same anatomical area, such as the thighs, because insulin absorption varies in different parts of the body. If you don't compensate for the difference, you may throw your control off. When you inject in your abdomen, for example, it absorbs, according to a study, 86 percent more quickly than in your leg, and 30 percent more quickly than in your arm. You will achieve much more consistency in the effectiveness of your insulin without added concern about reactions or high sugar if you don't switch around from one area of your body to another.

If you want to inject your abdomen or arm, an area you probably do not usually use, you may have to reduce your dose by about 5 units unless your sugar is high and you want to take advantage of the greater absorption. If you aren't aware of the differences, you may have some unexpected reactions.

Just to confuse matters, it is important to remember that insulin absorption also increases if you inject in an area that is going to get immediate heavy exercise. So, if you are going to go biking, don't inject in your leg. If you'll be playing tennis, don't choose your racquet arm. Unless, of course, you have high sugar and want to bring it down in a hurry.

## Injecting the Insulin

Wipe the area with a piece of cotton soaked in alcohol, or a prepared alcohol swab. With one hand, pinch a large fold of flesh between your thumb and forefinger at least three inches apart. Or, to inject into your upper arm, lean against a door to push your flesh up.

With the other hand, pick up the syringe like a pencil or a dart. Push the needle quickly and firmly into the skin, straight in perpendicular to the skin. (For small children and very thin people, a 45-degree angle may be better.) Pull back slightly on the plunger with the needle in place. If blood appears at the tip of the syringe, you have hit a small blood vessel. This isn't dangerous but may cause bleeding and bruising. (There's no harm in continuing with the injection, however, rather than withdrawing the needle.) Try to take no longer than about five seconds for the whole job. Now release the pinch and press an alcohol pad next to the needle and pull it out.

To prevent the possibility of a clogged needle, always inject the insulin *quickly* after pushing in the needle. But if the needle does clog, withdraw it and *write down* the number of units you have injected (your original dose minus the number of units remaining in the syringe). Take a new syringe and inject *only* the amount you still need to complete your full dose.

Occasionally you may notice that a little insulin squirts out when you make your injection and you don't know how many units you have lost. Or, as you take the needle out, there is more than the usual flow of blood, and again, you wonder if you have lost insulin. *Never* give yourself another injection. Probably you have not lost much, so simply eat a little less, and check your blood before lunch and dinner. If your sugar is high, you may need an extra dose (perhaps 4 to 5 units) of Regular insulin. Check with your doctor.

## IF YOUR VISION IS POOR

If you can't see the numbers on the syringe, you may be glad to know that you can buy special inexpensive products that magnify the syringe and its numbers. Others enable you to tell with your fingers when you have filled the syringe with the prescribed dose of insulin. One device, for example, clicks as it counts off a certain number of units of insulin; another has gauges to measure units, while yet another measures a preset dose. Most of the devices are available from The Lighthouse (800-334-5497).

## STORING YOUR INSULIN

If you don't like to inject cold insulin, you needn't refrigerate the bottle in use if you finish it within a month. After a month, discard it. But try to keep it in a cool, dim place, and be careful not to subject it to extreme temperatures.

Store your extra, unopened bottles or insulin cartridges in the refrigerator, but *never* put them in the freezer. Freezing destroys the insulin's potency. If a bottle freezes, throw it out. Never let it get very hot either. Don't keep it in your car's glove compartment, or on a windowsill in the sun or near the oven.

Insulin is marked with an expiration date. After that date, even an unopened bottle may start losing its strength. In an emergency, outdated insulin may be used until you have a new supply. It loses strength very slowly. Under ordinary circumstances, though, if you see yours is outdated, don't use it.

Regular insulin must be clear and colorless, just like water. If it becomes cloudy or discolored, don't use it. The other insulins should not become granular or clumped or form a deposit of solid particles. If they do, do not use them.

## INSULIN PUMPS

Insulin pumps have wrought near-miracles for many diabetics who have never before been able to achieve tight blood-sugar control. These people include some type 1 diabetics who are exceedingly hard to regulate, some pregnant women, and brittle diabetics who swing rapidly from one extreme of blood sugar to the other. Most people can do very well on their own, but occasionally the pump completely changes a poorly controlled diabetic's life.

The pump is a small, lightweight computerized battery-powered device about the size of a beeper that can worn on your belt or carried in your pocket. It is programmed by you and your doctor to deliver a steady, measured amount of Regular insulin around the clock. It will also send a surge (bolus) of insulin when you give it a special command before meals and large snacks. All this is done by way of an infusion set, a long thin tube with a needle or catheter at the end that is inserted under your skin in rotated sites, usually on the ab-

domen. Depending on your needs, the pump can hold a one-
or two-day supply of insulin.

The pump simulates as closely as possible the insulin output of a normal pancreas in response to food and has been responsible for impressive results for some diabetics who never
imagined they could do so well.

Although the pump should be worn day and night, it's possible to remove it for an hour or so for lovemaking, a bath, or
a very special occasion.

On the other hand, the pump is not without problems. It is
awkward. It can cause infections at the infusion sites. The
tubes can get clogged and the mechanism can fail, so it should
be checked regularly. If you suspect trouble, call the 24-hour
toll-free number found on the back of the device for technical
advice. Meanwhile, test your blood glucose and inject your
insulin yourself with a syringe, if necessary.

Since pumps are expensive and monthly maintenance can
be high, some health insurance policies refuse to cover them.
The pumps require careful training, supervision, and practice
to use correctly. Blood sugar must be monitored at least four
times a day.

If you are an orderly, organized, and perhaps compulsive
person, the pump could be your answer. But for most people,
it is probably best to stick to the rules and do without one.

## THE IMPLANTABLE PUMP

A more sophisticated kind of insulin-delivery system just
coming into use is the implantable pump which is surgically
implanted under the skin and injects insulin directly into the
abdominal cavity. Like the external pump, this device does
not monitor or respond to blood-glucose levels, but is programmed ahead of time by the doctor to release a low but
constant flow of insulin throughout the day. At mealtimes,
you use a remote-control device to direct the pump to release
additional doses. Every four to twelve weeks, the pump's

reservoir is refilled with insulin by the doctor. Not cheap, the implantable device seems to mimic more closely the natural production of insulin by the body.

Yet another device designed to deliver insulin automatically is in development, this one using a closed-loop feedback system that could eventually become a real substitute for one's own pancreas. It consists of a sensor that continuously monitors your blood-glucose level and a pump that releases the appropriate amounts of insulin in response. However, the device is at present the size of a television set and therefore not exactly handy.

## MIXED AND SPLIT DOSES

Most diabetics today take a mixed dose of Regular and Intermediate-acting insulin at the same time, using one injection or more a day. The Regular insulin has a short action span and works quickly. The Intermediate-acting insulin works over a longer period of time.

Many people get along very well with just one injection a day but others do much better with a split dose, taking most of their daily amount (perhaps 75 percent) in the morning and the rest in another injection before dinner or bed. This allows a fairly close approximation of the normal physiological pattern, smoothing out the peaks and valleys of available insulin.

If you tend to have late-morning or afternoon insulin reactions with only one daily injection, your doctor will undoubtedly recommend the split dose, probably combining Regular and Intermediate insulin each time. If you can't eat your meals at set times, you may do best with NPH at night and Regular before meals.

## MULTIPLE INJECTIONS

To get optimum control, even more than two shots a day are required by some people. Obviously, if you can do well without multiple injections you won't want them, because this regime is not easy or fun. But it is well worth the bother if this is the only way you can maintain good control. Your gains are far greater than your efforts. On the other hand, some compulsive patients insist on checking their blood sugar as often as five or six or seven times a day and taking insulin accordingly. This is not necessary. No need to become so obsessed by your diabetes that it's all you think about.

Of course, most insulin-taking diabetics must take multiple injections during stress periods such as an illness or a pregnancy.

Whether you take the multiple injections on a daily basis or only temporarily, your insulin intake must be adjusted according to your test results. If, for example, you are taking a combination of Regular and Intermediate-acting insulin and get these results, you must make these changes:

| Before Breakfast | Before Lunch | Before Dinner | Before Bed | Add |
|---|---|---|---|---|
| Under 150 | Over 150 | Under 150 | Under 150 | Add more units of Regular insulin in the morning. |
| Under 150 | Over 150 | Over 150 | Over 150 | Increase Intermediate insulin (and bedtime snack if you get nighttime reactions). |
| Under 150 | Under 150 | Under 150 | Over 150 | Add Regular insulin before dinner or reduce carbohydrates at dinner. |
| Over 150 | Under 150 | Under 150 | Over 150 | Add Regular and Intermediate-acting or Regular alone before dinner. |
| Over 150 | Under 150 | Under 150 | Under 150 | Reduce bedtime snack or take small amount of Intermediate insulin at bedtime. |

## HOW TO DISPOSE OF USED SYRINGES AND NEEDLES

Never toss used syringes, needles, or lancets directly into the trash can because they are medical waste that has had contact with human blood. You can buy an inexpensive piece of equipment called a safe-clip that clips, catches, and contains the needles. Or place these "sharps" in an opaque puncture-proof hard plastic container with a tight-fitting screw top. Don't use glass because it can break. Never use aluminum cans because they can bend. Label the container. Seal it with heavy-duty tape, and put it in the garbage—*never* in a recycling bin, because it could pose a danger to recycling workers and/or cause problems in the recycling process.

Your community may have special laws about syringe and needle disposal, so check with your local health department.

## "OOPS! I'VE MADE A MISTAKE!"

It happens to everyone. You forget to take your insulin, you take too much, or get the amounts mixed up. Don't panic. Here is how to deal with your mistakes:

### Forgetting to Take Your Insulin

Suppose you get up in the morning, eat your breakfast, go to work or school and suddenly in the middle of the day you realize you didn't take your morning shot.

Now you must take more Regular (because you are behind in the insulin you need) and less longer-acting (because there is less time before your next morning shot).

Let's suppose you normally take 10 Regular and 30 Intermediate-acting in the morning. If it is now about 11 A.M., take your injection, using slightly less but close to your normal dose. If you don't realize your omission until 3:30 in the afternoon and you start having symptoms of high sugar, take 20 Regular and 20 Intermediate. You need quicker action (therefore the increased Regular) over a shorter time span (therefore the decreased Intermediate).

Suppose you are at work or school or far from home when you realize you haven't taken your insulin. Call a doctor in the area and arrange to go to the office for a shot. Or go to the emergency room at the local hospital, telling the admitting clerk you cannot sit around waiting but must be attended to quickly. A third possibility is to get the name and telephone number of a drugstore in the area and then ask your own doctor to call this pharmacy and prescribe a syringe and insulin for you.

## Taking a Double Dose

Suppose you take your shot, have your breakfast, and give yourself another shot by mistake. Once in a while this won't hurt you if you eat enough to compensate for it—but don't make a habit of it. Meantime, have a field day. Have all those ice cream sodas, chocolate sundaes, coconut cakes you've been longing for. Space them out during the day and have a good snack before bed. Set your clock for 3 A.M. Get up and have another snack if your blood-sugar level is still low. The next morning, start your usual regime.

## Reversing Your Split Doses

A common error is to take what you normally take in the morning (the larger portion of your split dose) in the afternoon before dinner. In other words, suppose you normally take 10 Regular and 30 Intermediate in the morning, and 4 Regular and 10 Intermediate before dinner. Today you take your morning dose and then, before dinner, you unthinkingly take the same dose again, much more than you should at that hour. Again, eating is the answer. Eat more at dinner. Have a large bedtime snack and set your alarm clock for 3 A.M. Get up and check your blood-sugar level. If it is low, have some more goodies.

## PREPARING FOR AN EMERGENCY

*Always* have a bottle of Regular insulin stored in your refrigerator, even if you don't use it ordinarily. It will keep almost indefinitely though you should replace it when it becomes outdated. However, once it's opened, discard it after a month. Regular insulin is always used when you need quick action.

## INSULIN IN FOREIGN COUNTRIES

Insulin may be purchased all over the world and it is the same as you buy at home, whether or not it is made by an American manufacturer. Just be sure to buy the proper strength, or, if you cannot, also buy a syringe that corresponds to the strength you will be using (see Chapter 16).

## ARE YOU A "BRITTLE" DIABETIC?

A brittle diabetic is insulin-dependent, has extreme lack of control, with blood sugar that swings widely and rapidly from one extreme to the other, and so is in constant danger of insulin reaction on the one hand and acidosis on the other.

If you are a true brittle diabetic, you must follow all the rules very rigidly, checking your blood four times a day so you always know exactly where your sugar level stands. You should have a home glucose monitor (see the next chapter) so you can read your blood sugar in an instant. You may also be a candidate for an insulin pump.

Why you are unstable is a mystery in most cases, but some people are extremely sensitive to a difference of one or two units of insulin. Others, because of neuropathy, have stomachs that do not empty quickly and so glucose does not get into the bloodstream fast enough. Some have defects in their compensation mechanisms so the liver doesn't release sugar when it is needed. And perhaps there are other reasons we don't yet know about.

But, in most instances, brittle diabetics are not *really* brittle. They have simply never learned how to cope correctly with their condition. Perhaps their doctors have prescribed doses of insulin that are much too high. Then they eat too much to prevent reactions, thus raising their blood sugar way up, then take more insulin to bring it down, in a never-ending cycle. Perhaps they are not eating the correct diet, or have not tried taking insulin in split or multiple doses.

Or they may not know how to handle sick days, exercise days, or days of little activity.

Before you accept a diagnosis of "brittle," be sure you and your doctor have explored all the possibilities.

# *8*

# TESTING YOUR BLOOD SUGAR

Although there are many more enjoyable experiences in life, you must test your blood for its sugar level. Testing is a diabetic's best friend because it tells you how well your body is handling the sugar it both produces internally and processes from the food you eat. It is a simple and essential procedure. You don't have to love it, but you have to do it.

*All* diabetics—whether their diabetes is controlled by diet alone, oral agents, or insulin—should test *every day,* no matter how they feel.

Many diabetics insist they can *tell* when their sugar isn't normal. That's why they don't bother to make tests very often. If they feel "off," then they make a test. But the truth is, few people can detect sugar fluctuations unless those levels fall very low or rise very high. It is a rare person who will notice any true symptoms unless blood sugar is below about 40 mgs or above 400, and some people don't notice them until their sugar goes much higher than that.

Find out for yourself. Note down your feelings, decide whether you feel normal, high or low, then test your blood four times a day for a couple of weeks. Were you always correct? It is extremely doubtful that you were.

## WHY MUST YOU DO IT?

Why is testing important? Why, if you feel well, must you know your blood-sugar level? Because the effects of diabetes are cumulative, and it is well known today that consistently high or even moderately high sugar over a long period of time can help to bring about dire physical complications. It is very important that your sugar is consistently normal most of the time because high levels of blood sugar have an eventual deleterious effect on every organ of the body. You must also maintain a log of the test results so that glucose values can be tracked over time.

## GLYCOSURIA AND RENAL THRESHOLDS

Very few diabetics today measure their blood-sugar levels with urine tests, once the only way to do it. Blood tests are much more accurate and you should promptly switch to them even if you are an inveterate coward who can't bear the idea of sticking your finger. On the other hand, all diabetics must know how to test their urine for acetone (see Chapter 10).

Glycosuria is sugar "spilled" into the urine, and this sugar is what is measured when you make a urine test. The nondiabetic rarely spills any sugar because the normal body copes with incoming sugar by secreting enough insulin to cover it. Nor is a nondiabetic's blood sugar rarely higher than about 150 mgs percent. In diabetics, however, blood sugar can rise to phenomenal heights if it is not controlled by enough insulin.

There is one hitch to urine testing, and that is your individual renal threshold. The renal threshold determines how much sugar there is in your bloodstream before it spills out into the urine. Below a certain amount (different for everyone), the blood sugar is not excreted in the urine but is passed along to other parts of the body. Normally, blood sugar must be between 150 and 180 mgs percent before you spill.

Some, usually elderly, people have high thresholds. Blood sugar may be 220 mgs or more before it passes into the urine. Therefore they will have negative urine tests even when their sugar is extremely high. Others, usually children or teenagers, have low renal thresholds and will spill even though their sugar is not elevated above normal. And a few people lack the enzyme to return the sugar to the body and so sugar is spilled continually. This is called renal diabetes.

It is important then for you to know if your renal threshold is out of the normal range. If it is, it is more difficult to use urine tests as a sign of control because a high blood-sugar level may not cause a corresponding high value in the urine. That's why blood tests rather than urine tests will give you much more accurate readings of your blood sugar.

For a nondiabetic, fasting blood sugar is considered to be normal at about 70 to 100 mgs percent. One hour after a meal, 100 to 140 mgs is the usual normal range, but up to 175 may still be considered acceptable. Two hours after eating, blood sugar drops to about 80 to 120 mgs (but up to 145 mgs is still normal), then continues to fall until it reaches the fasting level again.

A diabetic's blood-sugar level often goes much higher than these levels, though it is important to aim for the normal range. You must try to keep your blood-sugar level at no more than 140 mgs percent fasting, and no more than 200 mgs two hours after a meal. A consistent pattern of blood sugars above these levels does not bode well for your future well-being.

## HOW OFTEN SHOULD TESTS BE MADE?

You must test your sugar level at least once a day, whether you take medication or not. And you should keep a record of the results.

Diabetics who are controlled by diet alone and whose sugars are usually low can probably get along well with blood tests only once a day or even just a few times a week. The results will tell you whether your diet requires adjustment or whether you may require medication to keep your diabetes under control.

If you take oral hypoglycemic agents, a schedule of two tests a day—before breakfast and before dinner—will inform you about your control. If you are not doing well, then you must also test before lunch and bed until you see normal results once more. You, too, must adjust your diet so that the oral agents will be sufficient to help you produce or utilize enough of your own insulin to compensate for what you eat. If you cannot do that, you may have to increase your dose, switch to another kind of oral medication, or graduate to insulin injections.

If you take insulin, then tests must be made at least three times a day—before breakfast, dinner, and bed. In times of stress, add a fourth test, before lunch. There's rarely a need to do it more often than that.

Each test gives you a report on the action of your medication vs. your food consumption and exercise during the immediately preceding period of time.

*No matter what kind of diabetic you are,* you must make at least four tests a day if you:

Have an infection, even a cold.

Feel nauseated or weak or have diarrhea.

Lose weight.

Are very thirsty or urinate frequently.

See any unusual pattern to your test results.


## KEEP RECORDS

Isolated test results won't tell you or your doctor very much, except that *at this moment* your blood sugar is high or low. But if you write down the results after each test, you will be able to detect a pattern to your blood-sugar levels and can then correct for any aberrations. An isolated high or low result isn't very important, but consistent highs or lows will tell you and the doctor that a change must be made. Your diet, your medication, or your activity may require adjustments, or an undiagnosed illness may need treatment.

Write your test results in a notebook, and make short notations about how you feel, whether you are ill, tired, stressed, if you have overindulged in food, underindulged in exercise, had a bad night's sleep, suffered an emotional high or low, etc.

Read over your accumulated test results once or twice a week to see if there are any recurring patterns of abnormal readings of high or low sugar levels, so you can make your own adjustments or discuss your situation with your doctor.

## IF YOU ARE SICK

Make tests at least four times a day, and test for acetone if your sugar is high. Talk to your doctor *at least once a day* for instructions about medication based on that day's test results (see Chapter 12).

## TESTING YOUR URINE

If you are among the few diabetics who still test their urine for sugar, here's how to do it. Just keep in mind that testing your blood provides much more accurate results and should be the method you use.

Unless you are instructed otherwise, always make your morning test with a *second-voided* urine specimen. This means that you urinate after arising and discard the urine, drink a glass of water, then test a second specimen passed 30 minutes later. The urine you have collected throughout the night is a mixed bag; it contains sugar that may have arrived in your bladder at any time since you went to bed. The second voiding will provide you with urine that will reflect the last few hours.

To make tests later in the day, the same rule applies. It is best to urinate about an hour before a meal, discard the urine, drink a glass of water, and test a second specimen in half an hour or an hour. This specimen won't hold the sugar that forms the first few hours after a meal and so is more likely to reflect your current blood-sugar state.

Use Keto-Diastix to read the glucose level of your urine. These strips have two squares at one end of the strip, one to indicate acetone, the other to indicate sugar. At this moment, you are interested in your sugar reading. Dip the strip in the urine. Wait 15 seconds, then compare the sugar square with the chart that comes with the strips. It is blue when your sugar is low, turns shades of green as it goes higher, and brown when it is way up there.

| Color | Percent sugar | Level |
|---|---|---|
| Blue | 0 | 0 |
| Light green | ⅒% | Trace |
| Dark green | ¼% | 1+ |
| Olive green | ½% | 2+ |
| Light brown | 1% | 3+ |
| Dark brown | 2% | 4+ |

## TESTING FOR ACETONE

Whenever you get a high sugar reading, it is imperative to test for the presence of acetones (or ketones) because, if you are producing these acids as a result of burning fat instead of carbohydrate, you *must* know it and correct it promptly. If you don't, you are setting forth on a short road to acidosis and plenty of trouble. If your urine shows acetone as well as high sugar, *check with your doctor without delay* about what to do. Perhaps you'll be told to take more medication immediately or wait to see if the acetone decreases. Test for it every two to four hours until it is completely gone. See Chapter 10 for more details.

When you test for acetone, use Keto-Diastix, little plastic strips that contain two test areas, one for sugar and the other for acetone. Dip the strip in the urine. Wait 15 seconds, then compare the acetone square with the chart. If you have acetone, the square will turn lavender or purple.

| Color | Amount of Acetone |
|---|---|
| No change | None |
| Lavender | Small amount |
| Light purple | Moderate amount |
| Dark purple | Large amount |

If your finger-stick blood test indicates that your blood sugar is low or normal although your acetone is high, that means you are not consuming enough carbohydrate. Nothing to worry about. Just correct your eating habits.

But, if your sugar is *high* and your acetone is *also high,* that's serious. Call your doctor because you will require more insulin than usual.

## HOME BLOOD-TESTING METHODS

Blood testing, which has almost totally replaced urine testing, gives you very specific blood-sugar readings. It tells you where you are *right now,* eliminating the time lag that is inevitable with urine testing.

Blood tests are especially essential if you are sick, if you are a type 1 diabetic who finds it hard to maintain control, or a brittle diabetic who needs constant insulin adjustment, or if you are pregnant.

They are also useful to people who want to check the effect of certain foods on their blood sugars. For example, if you wonder if a scoop of ice cream, or an apple, or crackers, will raise your blood sugar far out of bounds, check your sugar two hours after you have eaten them. If your blood is not abnormally elevated, you are home free (provided you have a normal renal threshold).

Because there's no immediate clinical reason to make any kind of blood-glucose tests unless you are prepared to respond to the information they give you, you must know how to adjust your medication, food, and exercise accordingly. This takes study, experience, and motivation, after a thorough discussion with your doctor.

## HOW TO TEST YOUR BLOOD

It's astonishing—or maybe it isn't—how many people are afraid to prick their fingers to get the necessary drop of blood for testing. But after you have done it a few times, you will see it isn't really traumatic. Besides, help is here for those of faint heart. In place of a lancet (which you can buy in disposable form), you may wish to use an Autolet or Penlet. These spring-action devices release a lancet and need only to be pressed against your finger or other sites to prick it automatically. Most patients say this is almost painless.

Now, to get that drop of blood: Swab your finger with alcohol and let it dry. Press your thumb just under the tip of the finger to be used until the fingertip turns red. With your lancet or autolet, make a small prick and squeeze out a large drop of blood. Drop the blood onto your test strip.

You can prick any part of your fingertips but you will feel it least if you use the sides of the finger pads, because there are fewer nerve endings there. The thumb and the fourth finger are the least sensitive.

If you hate to prick your fingers, take heart. Now you can take blood from other parts of your body, such as your leg, arm, or hand, with new lancing devices; for example, Vaculance and Freestyle.

## TESTING WITH A STRIP

Now, to see how much glucose is circulating in your bloodstream at this moment, you may choose to use chemically treated test strips such as Chemstrip bG. Keep in mind that this method gives you only a rough indication of your sugar level, nowhere near as accurate as the readings you get with a blood-glucose meter. Draw a drop of blood and place it on a strip. Wait 60 seconds, wipe the blood off with dry cotton, wait another 60 seconds. Compare the color with the guide on the container.

If the reading is more than 240 mgs percent, wait one more minute. It may move higher.

Even if you usually measure your blood glucose with a reflectance meter, you should know how to use these simple strips in case your machine malfunctions and you haven't been able to reach the manufacturer for technical advice. Better yet, have a second meter in reserve. They are not expensive.

## BLOOD-GLUCOSE METERS

For much more accurate readings of your blood sugar than you can get with a strip, use an electronic blood-glucose meter. Small enough to fit in your pocket, the meters are very simple to use. You place a drop of blood on a small test strip treated with an enzyme that changes color when exposed to glucose. Then you insert the strip into a slot in the meter, which then calculates and provides a digital readout of the value of your blood glucose.

There are so many varieties of meters available today, with more coming along every year, that you should discuss their merits with your physician before you make a choice. You should also check out the recommendations of the American Diabetes Association. Some meters are easier to use than others or perform tasks that the others don't, such as storing and recalling your last ten to fifty results. Some require smaller drops of blood, while others display the results more visibly. Important for many people, some meter strips will suck up a small amount of blood so you won't need a whole drop or allow you to simply smear the blood on.

Be sure to get detailed directions on how to use your meter and then remember to follow them carefully. Test the meter at least once a month according to the manufacturer's instructions; recalibrate it when you open a new package of strips; don't use strips that are outdated or have changed color; keep the meter scrupulously clean; check its accuracy periodically by comparing its readings with your doctor's findings.

Prices for meters vary widely. Check with your health insurance company to find out about reimbursement possibilities for both the meter and the strips.

Be aware that the meters may not always be accurate at very high altitudes or in extreme temperatures. Anemia, too, may affect their readings.

You may have heard about the meter that does not require blood but uses an infrared ray against the skin. However, this meter is many years away because of the cost of development and the problem of removing certain elements in the blood that give false readings. At the Mayo Clinic, researchers are developing a meter that uses tissue fluid instead of blood, which means you may soon be able to test blood glucose without sticking your finger.

## HbA1c: THE TEST THAT TELLS ALL

The blood-sugar tests we have been discussing give you important information about how good your control is today. The hemoglobin A1c test (HbA1c), a blood-sugar test made in a laboratory, tells how you have been doing for the last two or three months.

Because the hemoglobin A1c test tattles, reporting your past performance, it is especially important if you don't test often enough and tend to let your control slide. Or if you are one of those people who behave themselves for a week or so before each visit to the doctor but neglect their diabetes in between. Even though you know that consistently high sugars will cause disaster eventually, you may pay little attention until you get into trouble. This test, if it is made regularly, helps keep you on the path to righteousness.

Hemoglobin A1c is hemoglobin with glucose attached to it. Normally it is only a tiny part of your total hemoglobin supply. But when you have elevated blood sugar, the glucose tends to stick to the hemoglobin A that makes up 97.5 percent of your red blood cells. The more sugar in your blood, the more saturated the hemoglobin A becomes. Once the cells have glucose attached to them, the sugar remains there throughout their lifespan—about 120 days.

By measuring the A1c, your doctor will know your overall blood-sugar level for the last couple of months. A normal level ranges between 3.2 and 6.2 percent (equivalent to a blood-sugar level of 60 to 120 mgs), depending on the methods used by the laboratory. Keeping HbA1c to 8.1 percent or under helps you avoid diabetic complications in the future. A level higher than that indicates the need for prompt reform.

This test does not require fasting or repeated sampling, nor need it be done at any special time of day. It would be wise to have it made about every three months if you take oral agents or insulin. Meantime, don't forget your daily home tests.

NOTE: Occasionally, the hemoglobin A1c test fails to give accurate or useful results. The reason could be that it hasn't been made within the correct time limits or at a reliable laboratory; or the results could be skewed by wide swings in your blood-sugar levels just before undergoing the test. However, in almost all cases it is an excellent indication of your control during the last couple of months.

## FRUCTOSAMINE TEST: ANOTHER TATTLETALE

If you—and your doctor—don't want to wait three months between tests to find out if you've been keeping your blood sugars under good control, a fructosamine test is another way to keep you honest. This measures the amount of glucose that attaches not to hemoglobin but to a different substance in the blood. Unlike the A1c test which measures your blood glucose over the last two or three months, the fructosamine test issues a report on your control over the preceding two weeks. It is useful when you're making a change in your regime because you can tell right away whether your sugars are improving. It's useful for your doctor, who may suspect you've not been faithful to your diet. And, because the presence of abnormal hemoglobin does not alter its accuracy, it is useful for testing women with gestational diabetes (abnormal glucose tolerance that first appears during pregnancy, see Chapter 14).

In the future, when we know how to prevent glucose attachment to places where it shouldn't be, we will have to devise another test to measure diabetic control. In fact, in Japan, researchers are currently investigating 1,5-anhydroglucitol, a substance that can measure control without a protein such as hemoglobin attaching to glucose. And researchers at the California Institute of Technology are working on a glucose-sensing polymer that won't depend on current methods to detect recent control.

# INSULIN REACTIONS

**W**hen you are an insulin-taking diabetic, you quickly learn that you have a major concern which hardly anybody else ever worries about or knows exists. That's insulin reaction, very low blood sugar (hypoglycemia) caused by the presence of too much insulin in your bloodstream. Unless you are always spilling sugar (a bad idea), it is inevitable that you will have an occasional reaction, usually minor and easily handled. While reactions can hardly be described as delightful experiences, they are far healthier than having consistently high blood sugar, which in time can do inexorable damage to your body.

Besides, reactions can usually be avoided, and certainly minimized, by using your common sense.

In the nondiabetic, insulin is produced by the islet cells of the pancreas in response to the level of sugar in the bloodstream. The amount is always just enough to cover the sugar, and there is never too much. If the blood-glucose level falls too low, the liver releases more sugar from its standby stores, again just the right amount to do the job.

But diabetics who require exogenous insulin do not run on "automatic." They must try to match the amount of insulin they take with the blood sugar they *expect* to have. Sometimes, for various reasons, they have too much insulin in their bloodstream, and the blood-sugar level falls too low. When this happens, the brain and the central nervous system do not have the glucose they need for fuel and start to function less efficiently. The result is an insulin reaction.

## DIET THERAPY OR ORAL AGENTS

If you are a diabetic who is treated with diet alone, you will *never* have insulin reactions. If you take oral agents, there is a remote possibility of reactions under certain circumstances, but I have seen only a few in thirty-five years of practice. They occur in most cases only when there is a change in liver or kidney function, when overlapping medication is taken, or when the diabetic is elderly and frail, or is seriously ill and eats so poorly that he does not have an adequate store of glycogen ready to be released from the liver in emergencies. They can, however, be more severe than reactions from insulin, so take them seriously and report them to your doctor.

## WARNINGS AND SYMPTOMS

For an insulin-dependent diabetic, the possibility of a reaction begins when blood sugar falls below 40 or 50 mgs percent. Or when sugar takes a sudden nosedive, even if it goes from 400 to 200 mgs percent. The exact level as well as the symptoms vary for everyone.

Early warnings that a reaction is happening may include one or more of these feelings: weakness, sweating, headache, "butterflies" in the stomach, nausea, sudden hunger, anxiety, confusion, clumsiness, shakiness, pallor, palpitations, tingling of the lips, dizziness, a change in attitude, such as inappropriate laughing or crying. Most of these sensations result from the adrenaline (epinephrine) hormones your body pours into the bloodstream in an effort to raise your blood sugar.

Sometimes a headache is the only sign. Sometimes the feeling of being very tired for no particular reason is the sole warning signal. When this happens, don't go to sleep without checking to see if your blood sugar is low. If it is, you are probably starting to have a reaction.

Some people become very irritable, even hostile and aggressive, when their sugar is very low. Others find their vision becomes blurred.

If the reaction is allowed to continue, the symptoms may progress to slurred speech, mental confusion, dilated pupils, instability, and eventually to convulsions and loss of consciousness. A good rule for all insulin-taking diabetics: Before driving, count backward from 100 by sevens. If you can't do it, test your blood and, if necessary, take sugar immediately.

## WHAT CAUSES REACTIONS?

The low blood sugar that leads to a reaction is caused by just three things:

Taking too much insulin (sometimes by mistake).

Not eating when and what you should.

Exercising more than usual without compensating with extra calories or less insulin.

Reactions usually happen just before a meal, or when your insulin has its peak effect (see Chapter 7).

## ARE REACTIONS HARMFUL?

Most experts agree that mild reactions don't hurt you. And even severe reactions, with an extended state of unconsciousness and perhaps amnesia, almost never cause permanent damage.

## PREVENTION IS COMMON SENSE

If you know what triggers reactions, then you can almost always avoid them or head them off quickly.

• Always eat *on time* and eat *enough*. Never skip a meal unless you take less insulin. Don't forget your scheduled snacks.

• Be extremely careful when you measure out your insulin, double-checking to be sure you are taking the correct dose.

• If you are going to do more exercise than usual, eat more carbohydrate in preparation for it, or take less insulin, or both (see Chapter 5). Consult with your doctor to determine amounts. Before you set out to exercise, always test your blood for sugar. If it is low before you even begin, then you surely need to make adjustments.

Watch for reactions the day *after* heavy exercise, when your liver may still be depleted of its supply of extra glycogen. Your food, which normally would go into blood sugar, is now funneled into your liver to be stored, so you may need more food (or less insulin) in order to prevent hypoglycemia. Besides, you have increased your number of insulin receptor sites by exercising.

*During* your exercise, especially if it is strenuous and prolonged, it is quite possible you need some additional sugar. (Most people don't think of sex as exercise, but it is. Eat a snack before jumping into bed.)

• Sometimes, perhaps on a Saturday or Sunday, you may sleep late and skip breakfast. Since you are only going to eat two meals that day, be sure to take less insulin.

• An occasional reaction is nothing to be concerned about but if yours happen frequently, then you are doing something wrong. Usually the answer is that your insulin dosage is too high, or you are not eating enough at the right times. Review your diet and make sure you are eating a consistent number of calories that include the correct amount of carbohydrates. Check out your snacks. Are you getting enough carbohydrate and protein? There is *always* a reason for frequent reactions and you must find it.

Sometimes reactions tend to occur at the same time of day or night. Then you will know, *if you are eating correctly,* that your dose must be reevaluated and adjusted. Too much Regular insulin taken in the morning often causes reactions before lunch. Too much NPH or Lente may precipitate after-noon reactions when its action peaks. Your dose may be too high. Or you may do better with split amounts, giving you smaller but more frequent doses. Let your doctor know about your reactions and request that you review your dose, your diet, and your exercise together. If you continue to have prob-lems, perhaps you should go to another doctor, one whose specialty is diabetes.

## OTHER POSSIBILITIES

• The rate of absorption of the insulin you inject is affected by *where* you inject it. We know that the abdomen and arms usually have higher and faster absorption rates than the legs. If your reactions tend to occur after you have used these sites, maybe this is the reason. You can use this information to your advantage, not only to explain and prevent reactions, but to help you overcome high sugars more rapidly. When your sugar is high, injecting in your abdomen or arm can bring it down more rapidly.

• Pregnancy has a tremendous effect on your insulin needs (see Chapter 14), and you will probably require much less in-sulin in the first trimester (first 13 weeks) when the fetus and the placenta consume a lot of your circulating sugar and when you may not be eating as much as you usually do. This is a time when reactions are very common and can be severe. Dur-ing the rest of your pregnancy, you will undoubtedly require much *more* insulin than usual. But after the baby is born, your insulin needs will drop again—another time when you must be especially alert to the possibility of insulin reactions.

• The insulin requirements of menstruating women can be variable, too. Certain women need more or less insulin at some point during their cycle, usually the week *before* the period.

• Your emotional state can affect your need for more or less insulin. Although chronic stress seems to raise blood sugar, acute stress can lower it in a hurry, causing a reaction.

• Vomiting or diarrhea may deplete your body of the sugar it needs to function. You must get sugar somehow to avoid a reaction, so if you can't eat, drink regular (not diet) ginger ale for nourishment, take an antiemetic such as Compazine or Tigan in suppository form or by injection. And *immediately* call your doctor. You may need intravenous glucose if nothing else does the job (see Chapter 12). Be aware that one out of about 500 people gets an adverse reaction to Compazine.

• Too much alcohol consumption, too, can be the reason for insulin reactions, because it inhibits the release of glucose from the liver when you need it. Not only that, it may make you forget to eat on time.

• Certain drugs can have an effect on your insulin requirements. For example, beta blockers such as Inderal, Lopressor, or Tenormin, prescribed for hypertension, can mask the reactions so you won't be aware you're about to have one and you won't realize you need food.

• Some people, especially those who have had diabetes for many years, have "hypoglycemia unawareness"; in other words, they don't experience the usual warning signs heralding the onset of low blood sugar before lapsing into a full-fledged insulin reaction. If you are among those who don't realize your glucose level is dropping, be sure to cover yourself by testing your blood frequently.

• A caution for sauna devotees: A study has found that a sauna following your insulin injection can increase the absorption rate by 110 percent. So, have your sauna *after* a meal or snack, take along some carbohydrate, and since you won't be wearing your clothes or carrying your wallet card, be sure to wear your ID bracelet or necklace.

• Reactions can cause blurred vision and dizziness, so take special care when you're driving or operating machinery. Be sure your blood sugar isn't too low before you start, and have a snack every half hour or so if you stay at it for a long time. Remember the suggestion of counting backward from 100 by sevens.

• Hot or very cold weather also seem to affect some people's sugar metabolism because more energy is expended, especially when the extreme temperatures are combined with exercise. Be on the alert for reactions.

## NIGHTTIME REACTIONS

Many people, especially before their insulin dosage is adjusted properly, have reactions during the night or in the early morning. If this is the case with you, you should always, without fail, remember to eat a snack before bedtime. If there is no reason to suspect the hypoglycemia is caused by more exercise than usual that day or less food than you normally consume, *then your answer lies in your insulin dose.* You are taking too much Intermediate- or long-acting insulin in the morning. The doctor may suggest decreasing it by about 4 units to see if the nighttime reactions stop. If your daytime sugars go higher as a result, then a small amount of Regular insulin can be added to the syringe in the morning. Make changes in your dose only after consulting your doctor.

## KNOW YOUR BLOOD SUGAR

Diabetics who take insulin must test their blood a few times a day. If you keep a record of your sugars, you will be able to tell if there is a pattern to your episodes of hypoglycemia. You'll know if they seem to be caused by specific happenings in your life. You will also know when you must eat more or take less insulin so you won't have reactions.

When you know exactly where your blood sugar stands at any given moment, you can start to plan small adjustments in your eating or insulin schedules as needed.

## REACT TO A REACTION *FAST*

If you suspect you are beginning to have a reaction, don't wait around to see what's going to happen. Don't fight it. Do something right *now*. You may not have much time before you are in real trouble. Even if you are not sure that what you feel is a reaction, even if you think perhaps these symptoms may be caused by high sugar rather than low and you don't have the time or the facilities to test your blood sugar immediately, take preventive measures at once. In this case, better safe than sorry really applies.

Treatment at this stage is easy. Eat something. If the reaction is mild, some carbohydrate and protein (perhaps a glass of milk and some crackers) is sufficient. If it seems more pronounced or you tend to have reactions that come upon you quickly, take rapidly absorbed sugar: 2 teaspoons of granulated sugar—plain or dissolved in a little water; 6 or 7 Lifesavers or hard candies; 4 ounces of orange juice or regular (not diet) soft drink; 2 teaspoons of honey or corn syrup; a handful of raisins; whatever is handy and appeals to you most.

Some diabetics carry sugar cubes, glucose tablets, or little tubes of "Instant Glucose" with them. This is 25 grams of concentrated sugar that can be squeezed right into your mouth and absorbs very quickly. Or tubes of cake icing straight from the grocery store.

Don't overshoot the mark and take so much sugar that you will pay for it later in high blood sugar. You need 10 or 15 or, at most, 20 grams of sugar. After you have taken the sugar, *wait*. It takes 10 or 15 minutes for it to be absorbed into the bloodstream and reach your brain. If you don't start to feel better after 15 minutes, eat more.

Some people are so frightened of reactions that they start eating and keep on eating until the feelings have passed. By then they have so overdosed that it takes them days to get their blood sugar down to normal again. It is like killing a fly with a .22 rifle. Most effective in preventing rebound high sugars is a glass of milk with two crackers. Wait 15 minutes and repeat if necessary.

Obviously, the fuel you may need in a hurry must always be readily available to you. Carry some supplies in your pocket or handbag at all times, in the car's glove compartment, your suitcase, the desk drawer. One man keeps his in the top of his sock when he runs; another ties a little bag of sugar packets to his belt. No matter where you stash it, your emergency supplies must literally be at hand.

Important: Make a frequent check on your cache of sweets. Somebody else may have eaten them! Or perhaps you used them and forgot to stock up again.

## BACK TO YOUR NORMAL SCHEDULE

After you have taken extra food in response to a reaction, do not cut back on your regular eating plan. Forget you had it and eat as usual. That sugar is not to be calculated as part of your daily diet.

Your blood sugar will rebound within about an hour after treating a reaction with sugar, sometimes going as high as 200 or 300 mgs. Don't take extra insulin to counteract it, but test your blood again before your next meal.

## REACTIONS WITHOUT WARNING

You may be one of those diabetics who, after having had the disease for many years, tend to get reactions without any warning at all. If so, you must try even harder to avoid them. Test your blood four times a day. Be sure to have snacks at 10:30 A.M., 3:30 P.M., and before you go to bed, whether or not you think you need them. Include in your bedtime snack some protein (i.e., cheese or milk) as well as carbohydrate. During the night, your body will slowly convert that protein to usable carbohydrate.

## WHAT OTHER PEOPLE SHOULD KNOW

Just in case you ever have a severe reaction and can't respond to it yourself, train your family, responsible friends, and colleagues to know what to do. If you are in school, your teachers should know. Tell them that if you are conscious, they should give you the quickly absorbed sweets described on page 149, even if you object. Your low sugar when you have a reaction may make you stubborn!

If you are unconscious, that is another story. Nothing should be forced into your mouth because you may aspirate it. Now you will require an injection of glucagon, a hormone produced by the pancreas that raises blood sugar in a hurry, and you will be wise to keep a glucagon emergency kit handy, too, especially if you are prone to sudden and severe reactions. It requires a prescription and is available at drugstores.

The glucagon comes, with instructions, in a kit. Your helper combines a vial of solution with a vial of powder and injects it anywhere under your skin. It is extremely rare that one injection does not solve the problem of extreme hypoglycemia. It will probably bring you around in about 10 minutes and now you can take sugar by mouth. But if you don't respond, a second shot will not be effective. You must be seen by a doctor immediately or taken to a hospital emergency room for intravenous glucose infusion or other treatment.

Be sure someone in your family and at school or work knows how to give glucagon injections. It is very simple and requires no medical knowledge or expertise.

## THE DIFFERENCE BETWEEN INSULIN REACTION AND ACIDOSIS

Because acidosis, which we will discuss in the next chapter, can also lead to coma, it is sometimes difficult for you or another layperson to know the difference when you begin to feel peculiar or actually pass out. When in doubt, however, treat yourself for a reaction if you haven't the time to take a test, because insulin shock can lay you out very quickly. Diabetic coma happens gradually.

The best indication of an insulin reaction is profuse sweating, as opposed to acidosis when you hardly sweat at all. In acidosis, even your tongue and your armpits, a heavy source of sweat glands, will be dry because you have lost so much water in excessive urination.

Of course, the best way to know whether your sugar is low or high is to make a quick blood test, if you have time.


## LABEL YOURSELF

Not only should you let everyone with whom you associate know you are a diabetic who may have reactions, but it is most important to wear or carry something that identifies you as a diabetic—a bracelet, a necklace, and/or a wallet card that explains who you are and what to do in emergencies. It will let people know how to act in an emergency, and will help keep you out of the local jail, where many diabetics land when their behavior or lack of consciousness is misinterpreted as overindulgence in alcoholic spirits.

As a precaution, carry identification with you that says you are a diabetic and explains what should be done for you in an emergency. A simple way to do this is to join MedicAlert (800–344–3226). For a small fee, you get a wallet card and a stainless-steel bracelet or neck chain engraved with your personal identification number, a 24-hour-a-day toll-free telephone number, and a brief description of your medical condition. Information about your treatment is kept on file and is available to you or medical personnel who may need it in an emergency. Included in the file are the names and telephone numbers of your physician and people to notify in an emergency and other relevant material.

# 10

# COPING WITH ACIDOSIS

Though the exclusive rights to insulin reactions belong almost entirely to diabetics who take insulin, this is not the case with acidosis or ketosis, at the other end of the blood-sugar spectrum. *No matter what kind of diabetic you are and whether or not you take insulin, you are not immune to this complication,* which is caused by too little insulin and too much sugar in your bloodstream.

*Any* diabetic can go into acidosis with continued poor control or a sudden stress such as an illness or injury. Not only that, but acidosis is not a benign complication. If it is allowed to progress into diabetic coma, it can endanger your health and even your life if it is untreated.

But acidosis has one virtue; it doesn't happen suddenly. It develops gradually, usually over a few days. Even in the case of some type 1 or brittle diabetics, it takes about 12 to 24 hours. High sugar and acetone will show up in your tests. This gives you time, if you are paying attention, to prevent serious consequences. If you make blood tests every day and have learned to recognize the symptoms, you will always know when you are in danger of acidosis and so you can take appropriate measures.

## WHAT IS ACIDOSIS?

Acidosis or ketosis is a condition that results from hyper-glycemia, too *much* sugar in the blood because of too little in-sulin. In most cases, when the body lacks sufficient insulin to metabolize sugar, it starts burning its own fat and protein tis-sue for fuel. This emergency fuel produces acetone and other ketones, fatty acids that are released into the bloodstream, changing its chemistry to an acid state.

If acidosis isn't checked, coma and eventually death are the end results. Acidosis is *serious*. Happily, the current emphasis on good control and frequent tests have made it a much less common event than it used to be.

## THE WARNING SIGNS

You must act quickly as soon as you notice any signs of aci-dosis. What are the signs?

When your blood sugar increases without enough insulin to handle it, you will have the same symptoms that may have led you to the doctor when your diabetes was diagnosed. You will start spilling sugar into your urine. You will have to urinate frequently as the body tries to rid itself of the sugar, and will soon become dehydrated and extremely thirsty. Your skin will be dry. Your tongue will be dry. You may start to lose weight, your vision may be dim or blurred. Your breath, because you are burning fat instead of carbohydrate, may smell fruity or sweet like peaches or violets or freshly mowed hay.

Now, if you still don't acknowledge what's going on and deal with it, you will start to feel nauseated and perhaps de-velop abdominal pains. These symptoms will progress to a flushed face, labored breathing, drowsiness, disorientation, and eventually loss of consciousness.

## WHAT CAUSES ACIDOSIS?

The most common causes of acidosis are omitting your insulin or oral hypoglycemic agent or having an infection. It can also be precipitated by poor control (whether or not you take insulin), incorrect diet, failing to watch your blood-sugar levels with the proper vigilance and then not responding to high sugars immediately. *Preventing and dealing with abnormal sugar is a diabetic's Number One job.*

Sometimes you may not realize you are raising your blood sugar by eating too much of certain foods. In the summertime, for example, every doctor sees diabetics who have gone off the deep end with excessive amounts of fruit juices or raw fruits that are on their diet plan but not in the quantity in which they are consumed.

Illness, especially infection, dramatically increases your need for insulin, and is frequently the reason for an episode of high sugar and acidosis. *Be sure to take your insulin or pills when you are sick,* even though you are eating less or not at all. The fact is, you probably will need even *more* insulin, a situation you can judge only by making tests at regular close intervals. See Chapter 12 on coping with sick days.

Certain medications, such as prednisone, Dilantin, and protease inhibitors, used to treat AIDS, can aggravate your diabetes, raising your blood sugar and causing you to require more insulin. These drugs can cause a condition usually seen only in elderly diabetics. It is called hyperosmolar neoketotic coma, with extremely high blood sugar but no acetone to tip you off in advance. So be sure your doctor takes your diabetes into account when prescribing any additional drugs. This advice applies to all diabetics, whether or not you take insulin.

Sometimes you may not be taking the right amount of insulin or oral agent; you can tell this from your test results and should report to your doctor. You may forget to take your medication, fail to get your proportions correct if you take split doses, use insulin whose potency has been affected by freezing or excessive heat.

But, no matter the reason for your high sugar and even if acidosis has already begun, you still have time to turn the tide.

By the way, don't take your pills with juice—it raises your blood sugar. Use water instead.

## WHAT YOU SHOULD DO NOW

• Call your doctor the minute your tests show high sugar and acetone, or high sugar and the symptoms of thirst and urination.

• Check your blood *every two hours* when you see acetone.

• Take additional Regular insulin every two hours, or as instructed by your doctor, if your tests are very high. If you cannot reach your doctor immediately, a safe dose of Regular insulin is 20 percent (one fifth) of your usual morning dose of Intermediate-acting insulin. For example, if you normally take 40 units of NPH or Lente in the morning, add ⅕ of 40 units—or 8 units—of *Regular* insulin. If you don't normally take insulin, your doctor may tell you to take 5 or 10 units of Regular insulin every two hours if your blood sugar is over 250 or so.

• Continue to make tests every two hours, and take additional Regular insulin if your tests show high sugar and acetone.

• Do *not* take extra insulin if your sugar is low even though your acetone is positive. If it is extremely low, under 100 mgs, do not take your Regular insulin but only your usual dose of Intermediate. This means the acetone has not been entirely washed out of the body (it may remain about 24 hours after the sugar has been regulated), or that you have not been eating at least 50 to 100 grams of carbohydrate a day. Now is the time to eat or drink carbohydrate to provide glucose for fuel instead of fat.

• Rest, do not exercise.

• Drink as much water as you can to replace what you have lost.

• Keep in close touch with your doctor. Don't be afraid that you're being a pest, because if you let yourself go into coma, you will be much more bother than you are now. Extreme acidosis requires that you go to the hospital for treatment.

• If your doctor recommends hospitalization, don't resist. Your sugar and acetone levels must be brought down to safety—fast.

## REMEMBER THE THREE "T'S"

If you keep on top of your diabetes, you will never reach a state of serious acidosis or coma. In my thirty-five-year practice, with patients of all ages and all degrees of intelligence, I have rarely had to admit patients into the hospital for diabetic coma. That's because of the stress on tight control and three rigid rules:

1. Test your blood at least once a day; every two hours if you have high sugar and acetone.

2. Telephone your doctor.

3. Take extra insulin if you need it.

# WORRIES, WORRIES, WORRIES: THE CHANCES OF DIABETIC COMPLICATIONS

If you live a good long life (and there's little reason today to expect you won't), you may eventually meet up with what is known as "diabetic complications." Diabetes is a metabolic condition with cumulative effects on the various systems of the body, so the longer you have it the more likely it is that you will have complications from it.

While that is true, there is strong evidence today that the incidence and severity of the complications are closely correlated with diabetic control. That's why you should know about these possible long-term effects right from the start, long before there is the slightest sign of them. It is vitally important, even crucial, to your future well-being to maintain your blood sugar at a normal or near-normal level as much of the time as you possibly can.

Black Americans, especially women, not only have a higher incidence of diabetes but also are much more likely to suffer serious complications.

## HIGH SUGAR TO BLAME

Consistently uncontrolled blood sugar causes diabetic complications. If you don't want to end up with long-term damage to almost every part of your body, you must be vigilant about your blood-glucose levels. Granted, that is not easy but it can be done.

In the largest diabetes study ever conducted, the Diabetes Control and Complications Trial (DCCT) studied 1,441 type 1 diabetics in the United States and Canada for 10 years, from 1983 to 1993. The results showed that keeping blood-sugar levels as close to normal as possible slows the onset and progression of eye, kidney, and nerve diseases caused by diabetes. In fact, any sustained lowering of blood sugar helps prevent complications.

Among the volunteers, intensive therapy (very tight sugar control) plus strict attention to diet and exercise reduced the risk for developing retinopathy by 76 percent. It prevented the development and slowed the progression of diabetic kidney disease by 50 percent; it lowered blood cholesterol by 35 percent, and diabetic neuropathy by 60 percent.

In another study, this time of 4,400 diabetics, those with blood-sugar levels consistently under 300 had 3 times less risk of complications after 15 years than those with higher levels. Those who kept their sugar below 255 had 20 times less risk. And for the volunteers with levels consistently below 120, the risk evaporated.

## TAKE VITAMIN E

We now know that vitamin E can be helpful in preventing complications, reducing changes in the eyes and the kidneys by increasing the blood flow. So, unless there are contraindications in your case, we recommend taking a daily dose of 800 to 1,000 I.U. of vitamin E.

## REDUCE YOUR CHOLESTEROL LEVEL

Lowering your cholesterol level can help protect your eyes, according to current theory, because it will reduce the amount of fatty deposits leaking from weakened capillaries into the retina.

## MORE WAYS TO AVOID TROUBLE

Many drugs are currently under investigation as possible deterrents to diabetic complications. The first is LY33531, a compound that has been shown in animal experiments to decrease microalbuminurea (PKC-B), albumin produced by the kidneys, and to increase retinal blood flow. Others include aminoguanadine, ALT 462, and ALT 480, medications that can decrease the deposition of amyloid, a substance that clogs the filters of the kidneys.

## THE OSTRICH SYNDROME

Unfortunately, many diabetic newcomers refuse to think about their unwelcome ailment, won't accept it, and succumb to the "ostrich syndrome." As long as they don't have insulin reactions too often or lapse into comas and land in the hospital with regularity, they think they are doing just fine. Meantime, they don't monitor their carbohydrate intake or check their blood, and the constant high level of sugar circulating throughout the tissues of their bodies is having its inexorable effect. This happens often with "mild" diabetics who, because they take little or no medication, think they needn't be concerned and test their blood very seldom.

While many diabetic complications can be adequately treated medically, it is obviously much better to avoid them in the first place if you can. The best way to do that is to remain as close as you can to ideal control, starting *early* in your life as a diabetic.

And, if you do begin to develop any of the typical complications, *get on their case promptly*. Picking them up early means avoiding many of the possible problems. If you wait until they have had a good start, reversing them may be difficult. Be sure your doctor watches for them and tests for them regularly. Don't be afraid to ask about them or to insist on the proper checkups. Report any signs or symptoms the minute you notice them.

To some degree, diabetes eventually affects all the organs and systems of the body. Many of the medical problems of diabetics are no different from those other people have, but occur more often and earlier. Some simply accelerate the natural normal aging process, especially in the large blood vessels and the connective tissue. But others are quite special to diabetes, and occur because of specific changes in the smaller blood vessels and nervous system.

Much depends on the length of time you have had diabetes, the age you were when diagnosed, your race and your gender, and whether or not you must take insulin. Obviously, if you live long enough—diabetics tend to live to a ripe old age today—you are susceptible to more chronic problems, especially when you have a systemic condition. Besides, the longer you have diabetes, the more chance you have of acquiring any of the complications associated with it.

The more you know about diabetes, the fewer problems you will have, because you will understand the importance of tight control. Here are the pertinent facts about this collection of possible long-term diabetic complications.

## HEART ATTACKS, STROKES, AND ARTERIOSCLEROSIS

Arteriosclerosis, narrowing of the large blood vessels, is to be expected by all of us as we grow older. Coronary heart disease is the single most common cause of death in the United States today. Diabetics certainly don't own exclusive rights to it, but they do comprise a disproportionate percentage of the population to have it. As a group, diabetics develop arteriosclerosis, especially in the heart, head, and legs, much more often and earlier—perhaps a decade or so—than nondiabetics. It's been estimated by the United States Public Health Service that, while cardiovascular disease accounts for death among 50 percent of the general population, it is the cause of death for 75 percent of diabetics, who are twice as likely to have coronary heart disease, twice as likely to have strokes, and five times as likely to have arterial disease of the extremities.

One of the reasons for this situation is that diabetics have a predisposition toward hyperlipidemia, an abnormally high amount of cholesterol circulating in the bloodstream rather than being stored. This leads to the accumulation of deposits of fatty substances on the inner walls of the major blood vessels. The thought today is that your genetic makeup, what you eat, and how efficient your insulin supply is, are all important factors.

People with diabetes tend to be overweight and to have high blood pressure, two conditions that can aggravate cardiovascular problems. Obesity requires extra blood supply to nourish the extra body tissue, and puts it own strain on the heart as well. High blood pressure means an obvious stress on all the blood vessels, including the heart.

## SO WHAT CAN YOU DO?

Since you know you have a tendency to develop cardiovascular complications earlier and more rapidly than other people, your job is to try to head them off. First, of course, as always, you must maintain excellent diabetic control, not just today and for a few days next month, but constantly. The less sugar circulating throughout your body the better.

If you are overweight, it is essential to lose weight. As you lose, you will see dramatic improvements in your blood cholesterol levels and—a most important feature—a drop in your blood pressure if it is high. Because high blood pressure always multiplies the risk of heart attack and stroke, you must bring it down with diet or, if necessary, medication.

Be sure your doctor is aware that you are diabetic. This may sound ridiculous—of course, your doctor knows—but if you use different doctors for different ailments, that may not be the case. Or he/she may forget for the moment.

## A BAD MATCH: DIABETES AND SMOKING

Smoking causes arterial spasms and is definitely a habit that must go. Diabetes and smoking combine to increase by many times the risk of heart disease. A diabetic, who already has a tendency toward coronary disease, needs to have everything going for him. Arterial spasms constrict the blood vessels, decreasing blood supply to the extremities—not a good idea, especially in your case. Besides, smoking may increase your chances of developing retinopathy and vision problems.

## WATCH YOUR CHOLESTEROL

Because there is little controversy today over cholesterol's effect on your arteries, it is an excellent idea to limit the amount of saturated fats you eat and to increase the proportion of polyunsaturated varieties. If your cholesterol level is elevated, there are medications that your doctor may prescribe to help bring the lipid levels down to normal.

Your cholesterol level can be evaluated by the amount of high-density lipoproteins (HDL) it contains vs. the amount of low-density lipoproteins (LDL). The more high-density you have, the less chance there is that you will develop arteriosclerosis after age fifty. Exercise has been found to increase HDL, and so has an alcoholic drink or two before dinner. If your cholesterol value is below 150, it is not important to know what your HDL level is. It won't be high enough to matter. And if your cholesterol exceeds 350, it's too high to bother separating out. At this point, your HDL level is rarely sufficient to protect you from arteriosclerosis. Between those two extremes, however, knowing your blood's HDL/LDL ratio is important.

## ARE REACTIONS HARMFUL?

If you already have arteriosclerosis, you should do your best to avoid insulin reactions. That's because severe reactions are thought to put additional stress on the already narrowed blood vessels supplying the heart or the brain. However, this isn't as important as doctors have thought in the past. In fear of shocks, they have often allowed their patients to consistently spill too much sugar. Today the thinking is that reactions do not pose a great danger and that it is much more important to control blood sugar closely, even with the risk of a few reactions. In the long run, tight control is best.

## GET YOUR EXERCISE

Next, exercise. Everyone's cardiovascular system benefits from regular exercise, especially exercise that gets the heart pumping and the lungs expanding. If you get enough (always under the supervision of your doctor), you can significantly lower your risk of heart attack. Exercise can slow your heart rate, lower your blood pressure, help burn up calories, cut down LDL levels, raise HDL, and as an added bonus, help keep your diabetes under control by allowing you to handle carbohydrates more efficiently.

## THE ASPIRIN TREATMENT

Researchers are currently evaluating the use of aspirin for vascular disease because of its anticlotting effect. In addition, research has shown that it sometimes lowers blood sugar.

The answers are not yet in. In the meantime, it won't hurt to take a baby aspirin (81 mgs) a day. Check with your physician first, however. If you have retinopathy associated with hemorrhaging, or a tendency toward bleeding ulcers, it is *not* a good idea to take even a baby aspirin regularly.

## THE CHANCES OF EYE PROBLEMS

There was a time, not long ago, when all diabetics had a good chance of developing serious vision problems, but that has drastically changed in recent years. Though it is true that diabetes is still a leading cause of blindness, there is a 90-percent-or-better chance it's not going to happen to you. And the odds are improving in your favor every day because of new research and treatments.

Today we have excellent methods of coping with the typical diabetic eye changes. And we know that, with good diabetic control, especially in the first five years, you are much less likely to develop eventual difficulties. There are exceptions to every rule, of course, but, in general, people whose blood sugars are kept consistently below a certain level tend to show many fewer complications of all kinds.

Type 2 diabetics are not as likely to develop serious eye changes as those who have type 1 that usually strikes in childhood; black people are in a higher risk category; and people treated by diet alone or oral agents have less chance of eye complications than those who are dependent on insulin.

Nine out of ten diabetics eventually show some vascular changes in their retinas, the linings of the backs of the eyes where light is received and then sent to the brain for interpretation. Called background retinopathy, these early changes usually appear and then stay pretty much as they are, or sometimes clear up spontaneously and cause no problems with vision. Of the 90 percent of those diabetics who develop background retinopathy, only about 80 percent have vision problems and just one in five will progress to the next set of complications called proliferative retinopathy or retinitis proliferans. This is a more precarious situation, but even among people in this group, blindness can, in most cases, be prevented.

So, while this is definitely a concern, it is not inevitable and it gives you excellent reason to keep your blood-sugar levels within acceptable boundaries. Temporary lapses into high levels, which happen to everyone, aren't what we are talking about. It is the consistent lack of tight control that is much more likely to cause trouble later in your life.

You, as a diabetic, are also at risk for other eye diseases. For example, you are nearly twice as likely to get glaucoma as other adults, and this risk increases the longer you've had diabetes. Cataracts, too, are twice as prevalent among diabetics and tend to develop at an earlier age.

## WHAT IS BACKGROUND RETINOPATHY?

The retina is nourished by a network of tiny capillaries. After many years of diabetes, the walls or the basement membranes of these blood vessels become damaged, cutting down the oxygen supply to the eyes. They may then become weakened and form little bulges called microaneurysms. These, like any balloons, tend to have fragile walls and may leak serum inside the retina, sometimes causing macular edema—swelling from the leaking fluid. Sometimes, too, the tiny capillaries rupture and little hemorrhages occur in the backs of the eyes.

The doctor who examines your eyes looks for these microaneurysms, which show up as red dots, as well as small collections of soft, cottony or yellowish fatty materials which are actually cholesterol deposits and are called exudates. If you have them, you have background retinopathy, which does not mean things will get worse. This will probably become merely a chronic condition, which your diabetologist and ophthalmologist must check periodically. You probably will not even be aware of it and it will not affect your vision unless it occurs around the macula, a very small area responsible for your central vision.

## WHAT'S TO BE DONE ABOUT IT?

The very first thing you can do about retinopathy and your diabetes is to stop denying the truth. If you don't maintain very good control over your blood-sugar levels, you are issuing an invitation to a great many problems. Numerous studies have conclusively shown that sugar levels are closely linked with eye changes, all of them pointing to the importance of keeping the sugar within the normal range (below 140 mgs fasting and below 200 mgs two hours after eating), therefore keeping your HbA1c below 8.2 percent.

This is not to say that maintaining perfect control (which is impossible anyway) over many years will absolutely ward off eye complications. Some people take excellent care of themselves and keep their blood sugars very close to normal, yet still develop retinopathy, while others who are wildly out of control never have it. But, as a rule, the majority of diabetics who maintain good control will not have retinopathy, while the majority of those who do not monitor their sugar levels carefully will develop eye complications. This includes *all* diabetics on insulin, oral agents, or even diet alone.

The second thing you can do if you have background retinopathy is to be sure your blood pressure is within the normal range. Hypertension, even without diabetes, can cause retinopathy because the little blood vessels in the eyes are under stress. The combination of the two ailments obviously is undesirable. And, since smokers have a higher incidence of retinopathy, smoking, for this among many other reasons, is not acceptable for you as a diabetic.

## AN EYE CHECKUP EVERY THREE MONTHS

Be certain your physician examines your eyes at *every* visit (diabetics should see their doctors at least every three months), and *remind* the doctor, if necessary, to do so. If this chore doesn't seem very important to the person you have chosen as your physician, it might be a good idea to find another. The minute the doctor sees signs of retinopathy, you should promptly see an ophthalmologist (an M.D. with a specialty in ophthalmology—not an optician or an optometrist) and then return for checkups *at least* every six months.

In fact, you should see this specialist initially just after your diagnosis as a diabetic, especially if you have the type 2 variety of diabetes. You may have had asymptomatic diabetes for years before the diagnosis and it is an excellent idea to check out your eyes now.

Even without any eye changes, it's most important to see the ophthalmologist at least once a year. Do not wait for any sudden decreased vision or strange symptoms to make your first appointment, or even for your doctor to see evidence of microaneurysms. With the use of a special fluorescent dye, diabetic eye changes can be discovered by a specialist even earlier.

In addition to those regular visits to your ophthalmologist, it is an excellent idea to schedule an appointment with a retinal specialist at least every year after your fifth year as a diabetic. It's important to catch eye problems such as retinopathy and glaucoma as early as possible before your vision is impaired.

Meanwhile, be sure to take at least 800 to 1,000 I.U. of vitamin E every day and lower your cholesterol level if it is out of the normal range.

## PROLIFERATIVE RETINOPATHY EXPLAINED

Retinitis proliferans is more serious than background retinopathy and it's important to know that if treatment is going to be useful, you must start *early.* That means *right now,* just as soon as it is diagnosed. A study of 847 cases of retinitis proliferans at the Joslin Clinic, in which I was a principal investigator, showed that it takes 17.4 years, on average, for a youngster with type 1 diabetes who is going to have this condition to develop it; and 4.3 years, on the average, for a person over sixty. Your doctor should be aware of the natural history of this complication.

Only about 40 percent of people who already have retinitis proliferans report to their physicians that they have noticed changes in vision or are experiencing symptoms like streaks or flashes. This means the other 60 percent with serious eye changes do not have the signals or are not acknowledging them. That is why it is vital for your doctor always to check the backs of your eyes.

Retinitis proliferans works like this: the capillaries along the inner surfaces of the retina start multiplying or proliferating, probably as a response to decreased oxygen supply to the eye. These new blood vessels try to bring more oxygen into the area, just as fire hoses bring water to a fire, but they are very fragile. They break easily and then may bleed into the retina and the vitreous, the gel-like substance that fills the eyeball. This makes the vitreous murky, preventing the passage of light from the lens to the retina. Fortunately, the blood is often reabsorbed spontaneously and the vitreous clears again.

In some cases of retinitis proliferans, the rapid growth of new and delicate blood vessels and the resulting bleeding stimulates the formation of fibrous scar tissue that may contract and cause a detached retina. Retinitis proliferans can also lead to a form of glaucoma that can be difficult to treat. All of this usually comes about quite slowly. If the proliferation happens only on the periphery of the retina and the vitreous isn't clouded, vision won't be seriously affected. But if it covers the central portion of the retina, if the retina starts to detach, or if the vitreous becomes opaque, then we have problems. But even then, we have some solutions.

## WHAT IS THE TREATMENT?

Several good treatments have been developed and perfected in recent years, with others on the way. One of these is photocoagulation, which involves the use of a laser aimed at the leaking or abnormally proliferating blood vessels. The beam, which is usually painless, destroys the unwanted fragile capillaries and seals them off, resulting in harmless scar tissue. The laser is also used to shoot pinpoint blasts around the periphery of leaky eye tissue, closing off these outer capillaries to decrease the eye's oxygen requirements. Now more of the available blood will go to the central and most important area of the retina. Sometimes, the laser beam is used to glue the retina back in place if it is detached or in danger of becoming detached. Photocoagulation has become a major tool of the ophthalmologist and often manages to stop retinal damage right in its tracks. Lasers can also treat diabetic glaucoma.

A procedure called *vitrectomy* is another important new treatment for eyes seriously affected by retinitis proliferans. If the vitreous inside the eyeball has become clouded with little bits of leaking blood, or if it has started to contract because of the bleeding and to pull on the retina, threatening to detach it, this technique may be employed to improve the situation. A special precision instrument is used to bore a tiny hole into the eye and suction out the stained vitreous, at the same time replacing it with clear saline solution. This procedure can not only eliminate the clouded vision, but it can also give the ophthalmologist an opportunity to see into your eyes and evaluate the usefulness of laser treatment.

## WILL VITAMIN C HELP?

Though vitamin C in combination with rutin was once widely prescribed for retinopathy, studies have shown that rutin isn't absorbed by the body at all, and the effectiveness of vitamin C as a way to strengthen the capillary walls is still being debated. In other words, nobody knows for sure whether it will help prevent retinopathy, or colds either for that matter. Our theory is, though, that it can't hurt to take about 500 mgs of C every day. The best that could happen is that it works; the worst is that it doesn't. Excess vitamin C is excreted in the urine.

## IS VITAMIN E THE ANSWER?

Vitamin E can help prevent the development of retinopathy, according to a recent study by Sven-Erik Bursell, Ph.D., of the Joslin Diabetes Center in Boston. Bursell found that diabetic patients have 16 percent less blood flow in the retina and that blood flow normalizes with the use of vitamin E supplements.

Because vitamin E, an antioxidant, does other good things as well, such as protect your arteries and your kidneys, we suggest you take up to 1,000 I.U. of this vitamin as a supplement every day.

## WHAT ABOUT MAGNESIUM?

A study comparing three groups of diabetics found the lowest amount of magnesium in those with the greatest degree of retinopathy. From this it has been theorized that supplements of magnesium salts may be beneficial. Again, we don't have the answer yet. Since magnesium can be found in such foods as meat, cereals, and nuts, you probably don't need a supplement.

## MY VISION IS BLURRY. IS THAT BAD?

Not necessarily. Your vision can be affected simply by your current blood-sugar level. If the level is high or fluctuating, your sight may be fuzzy, out of focus. It will clear up when you're once more under good control, though it may take anywhere from a few days to a few weeks. *Nevertheless, always go to your diabetic specialist when your vision changes in any way.*

Blurred vision is *expected* when your diabetes is first diagnosed and you are treated with insulin for the first time. After undergoing a week or two of insulin therapy and having your blood sugar go down to an acceptable level, you may find you cannot focus clearly. Don't panic. It will get better before long.

Probably the blurred vision occurs because, during the period of poor control and dehydration, the eyes gradually lost some of their fluid content as well as fluids from the rest of the body, altering their shape. In addition, the increased sugar content in the eyes' lenses may cause them to swell and alter their refraction of light. As both these factors swing back toward normal, you will notice the blurriness until you adjust once more.

By the way, be sure your sugar is in optimum control *before* you go to the ophthalmologist for new eyeglasses. If your sugar is high, your distance vision may be affected. If it is very low, your near vision may change. So new glasses that are fitted today may not be right for you tomorrow or next week. If you are a new diabetic, wait at least a month after you have been stabilized before going for a different prescription.

## WHAT CAUSES DOUBLE VISION?

Very low blood-sugar levels can temporarily produce double vision. If the two images persist, however, it may be due to infarction of a nerve of the eye muscles and an uneven pull of the muscles. If an eye is pulled off-center unilaterally, you will see two images, a decidedly unpleasant phenomenon. But don't worry, it disappears spontaneously within three to six weeks in just about every case, and all you'll need is an eye patch until it does.

## DO DIABETICS HAVE MORE CATARACTS?

They do. They also tend to get them at an earlier age and the progression is more rapid. Cataracts include both the "snowflake" metabolic variety that occasionally occurs in type 1 diabetics and the "senile" kind that is part of the normal aging process.

Treatment for cataracts is the same for everyone, though for diabetics the doctors may decide on surgery at a slightly earlier stage of development in order to have an opportunity to examine the back of the retina.

With cataract surgery, as with any other kind of operation, it is very important to be under optimum control when you have the procedure so that healing will be normal and infections more easily avoided.

A lens implant at the time of surgery will not interfere with laser treatment if you ever require it at a later time.

## DO DIABETICS HAVE MORE GLAUCOMA?

Yes, and the longer they have had diabetes, the greater the risk of developing it. It's important to catch glaucoma early so it can be treated with medications and/or laser or other forms of surgery before it impairs your vision. Glaucoma develops slowly and insidiously without any obvious symptoms. Half of those who have it don't even know it.

## ARE CONTACT LENSES SAFE?

There is no reason you cannot wear contact lenses if the outer surfaces of your eyes are in healthy condition. Be sure, however, to go to a reputable ophthalmologist who has extensive experience in fitting contacts. You may choose hard or soft lenses which are taken out every day, or left in for longer periods of time.

## SHOULD I WORRY ABOUT "FLOATERS"?

Floaters or "flying mice," as they have been dubbed, are little pieces of protein that you can see fleetingly as they float through the vitreous, the gel-like fluid within the eyeball. These are nothing to be concerned about unless they develop suddenly or are accompanied by flashes of light (in which case, see your ophthalmologist immediately). Most people have floaters, though diabetics seem to have them more often than others.

## THE EFFECTS OF MARIJUANA

Marijuana lowers the pressure within the eyeball, so it is theoretically possible that it may encourage bleeding of the fragile capillaries of the retina. This is a good reason, along with a few others, not to use it. It encourages a desire for sweets among some people, which diabetics can't afford, and tends to alter the sense of time. You may forget to eat on time and then have a serious insulin reaction.

## THE EFFECTS OF EXERCISE

Regular vigorous exercise helps to prevent retinopathy and other diabetic complications although you should never lift weights above your eye level if you are diabetic. But the story is quite different if you already have retinopathy. Now it's important *not* to raise your blood pressure, which can trigger more hemorrhaging of those tiny blood vessels in the backs of the eyes. Don't do anything strenuous without consulting your doctor, and don't even think of lifting weights.

## KIDNEY PROBLEMS

Because your two kidneys, located just to either side of your spine, are intricate filters with the important job of eliminating waste products from the blood while holding on to certain vital proteins, it is very important that they continue to function smoothly. Kidney complications, however, can be one of the problems that beset long-time diabetics, especially black diabetics, among whom chronic kidney problems due to this disease are almost three times greater than among white diabetics. This is because of a tendency for all of the blood vessels in the body to weaken and for the walls or basement membranes of the kidneys' complex network of capillaries to thicken and, at the same time, become too porous. These incredibly complicated filters then allow a loss of proteins—albumin and globulin—into the urine. Further progression can result in uremia and kidney failure, which can be treated only by dialysis or kidney transplants.

Other factors that can lead to kidney complications are high blood pressure and urinary infections, problems diabetics are prone to have. Pressure control is extremely important, and so is the early and vigorous treatment of infections.

And, as always, keep your diabetes under good control. There is solid evidence that kidney damage can be prevented or at least lessened by about half with strict control, and other indications that it might even be somewhat reversible.

In addition to tight control, ACE inhibitors such as captopril (brand name Capoten), a drug commonly used to treat high blood pressure, slow the progression to diabetic kidney failure if used early enough. They keep the kidneys healthier by inhibiting the production of an enzyme that makes blood vessels constrict. A three-year study published in 1993 found type 1 diabetics who take captopril have half the risk of dying or having their kidneys fail as those who don't. Other antihypertensive treatments may also slow the progression of kidney disease.

There's promise, too, of another mode of defense against kidney failure with the use of newer compounds such as aminoguanidine, glycosaminoglycans, and LY 33531, currently being tested. Used early on, they seem to help prevent "advance glycation end products," when glucose attaches to the kidneys, causing them to become waterlogged and thickened.

Don't forget to take your vitamin E every day!

## TESTING FOR EARLY KIDNEY PROBLEMS

The presence of microalbuminurea—small deposits of albumin in the urine—is a warning sign that you are at risk of developing kidney disease. A simple urine test that can detect these low levels of protein should be part of your regular checkups. The problem is that the usual urine tests can only detect a level of 300 mgs of albumin, and the first red flag for this disease may start at much lower levels, perhaps even at 30 mgs. When your doctor suspects trouble, more sophisticated testing is required.

By the way, some drugs such as ibuprofen may not be safe for people with kidney disease. Don't take *anything* without consulting your doctor.

## NEUROPATHY

Neuropathy, probably the most common as well as the strangest of all the possible diabetic complications, affects nerve function and isn't very well understood even today. Its symptoms can be mild and simply an annoyance, or they can make life pretty miserable. The only good thing about neuropathy is that its weird effects sometimes disappear or improve dramatically after a while. This can take from a couple of months to a couple of years.

Because neuropathy is nerve damage that interferes with the ability of the nerves to conduct messages and at times actually alters them, sometimes it results in outright severe pain, sometimes in tingling, a pins-and-needles sensation, burning, itching, or simply numbness. Occasionally there will be pain and numbness at the same time. These symptoms, which can show up in many parts of the body, come and go unpredictably, though for most people they tend to be decidedly worse at night. And they often confound the medical experts, who may diagnose them as something else.

Nobody knows just why neuropathy happens, but research indicates that the "sorbitol pathway" may be at the bottom of it. When sugar persistently circulates at high levels in the body tissues, certain enzymes turn the glucose into fructose, then into sorbitol. Sorbitol, a sugar that cannot return to its previous incarnations as glucose and fructose, causes damage to the nerve endings so they are unable to carry on their normal metabolism and consequently their normal function. Sorbitol taken by mouth, however, does not affect the nerves.

## WHERE NEUROPATHY STRIKES

Neuropathy most often affects the legs and feet, where it gives you pain or tingling, or the odd impression of walking on sand or pebbles. Often there's a *lack* of sensation, so it feels as if you are walking on wood or even on pillows or clouds. Some people say it feels as if their feet do not belong to them. Others have pain and lack of sensation at the very same time and some become extraordinarily sensitive to touch so that even the weight of sheets is a torment. The pain may be constant or intermittent, usually becoming much more troublesome at night. Often it occurs *only* at night, disappearing when the sun comes up. Cold, wet weather seems to aggravate it.

If you haven't much feeling in your feet, you will now have to be especially careful not to injure them without realizing it, and to keep an eye out for infections you can't feel. See Chapter 13 for a complete discussion of foot care.

If you have neuropathic pain, take comfort in the fact that it may get better in a few months. In fact, some specialists say the worse the pain, the faster it goes away, leaving some numbness in its place. Meantime, you may need painkillers or tranquilizers to help you sleep. Most physicians prescribe a tricyclic antidepressant such as Elavil or Desaryl, perhaps in combination with a mood elevator such as Prolixin so that narcotics can be avoided in the quest for a good night's sleep. This can be quite effective. A drug called Neurotonin is another choice. But Dilantin isn't recommended because it usually doesn't work and it decreases whatever insulin secretion you have, interfering with glucose metabolism if you are on oral agents or diet alone. Besides, Dilantin, as well as steroids—cortisone, for example—may lead to hyperosmolar coma, a condition in diabetics that can be even worse than the coma caused by acidosis.

## OTHER NEUROPATHIC HAUNTS

Though the feet are neuropathy's favorite targets, it can affect other parts of you too. Occasionally people find their hands become somewhat insensitive, almost as if they are wearing gloves. Sometimes the muscles of the hands diminish in size, or the muscles between the fingers become atrophied, making it difficult to use the hands for small movements such as buttoning a shirt.

Diabetics also sometimes develop a condition called Dupuytren's contracture. The tendons of the palm of the hand become thickened and shortened, hindering mobility. Surgery can correct these "frozen" hands.

Occasionally neuropathy affects the muscles of the eyes, causing double vision and perhaps sharp pain. The prognosis is usually excellent for double vision, with complete recovery within about six weeks.

The gastrointestinal tract is another part of the body that may be affected by this strange nerve damage peculiar to diabetes. The esophagus and stomach, as well as the intestines, may not contract with their usual vigor, with the result that they don't empty efficiently. The delay may affect your diabetic control by delaying the absorption of the food. Or it may cause bloating or perhaps nausea. It often helps to cut back on the fat in your diet and to take Reglan, a drug that speeds up intestinal peristalsis. For some people, other helpful drugs are Cisapride and Propulsid, taken half an hour before meals. Warning: breast tenderness may be a side effect.

Some people with intestinal neuropathy find they develop diarrhea at unpredictable moments, most often at night. Or they become severely constipated. About half of those with diabetic diarrhea respond well to antibiotics such as tetracycline, Flagyl, and especially erythromycin, which work on the intestinal bacteria. Other people get good results from anti-diarrhea medications such as Lomotil or codeine. The constipation usually responds to laxatives or stool softeners. Drugs such as Reglan to stimulate smooth muscle tissue may be helpful as well. Keep in mind that fatigue and stress have a poor effect on bowel problems.

The bladder may also be affected by this strange villain if the nerve damage interferes with its ability to contract, or with its owner's ability to sense when it is full and needs emptying. The urine may back up into the kidneys or the bladder may not empty completely, providing a happy home for bacteria and infections. Sometimes drugs such as Hytrin or Cardura can improve this organ's muscle tone and its ability to empty.

## URINARY PROBLEMS

Because constant urinary infections that may hang on stubbornly can eventually lead to serious kidney disfunction, all diabetics must be sure to watch closely for them. If you have any symptoms of an infection, such as burning, pain, or urgency, see your doctor immediately. Make certain you are given the proper tests to determine the right drugs to combat it, and that you stay on the drugs until the infection is totally destroyed. If you have a tendency to get infections, your doctor should check for them by examining your urine under a microscope at every examination (at least every three months) *whether or not* you have symptoms.

If you're a woman, make sure to drink a lot of water before and after sex to keep the infection rate down. And always wipe yourself from front to back.

If you notice you are not urinating very often and, when you do, you produce a less-than-expected amount, discuss this with your doctor, who may suggest that you urinate every few hours on schedule rather than wait for the urge, or may prescribe drugs to stimulate urination.

## NEUROPATHIC FOOT ULCERS

Because neuropathy often causes a lack of feeling on the bottoms of the feet, it's possible to develop sores, usually at pressure points, that you are unaware of. This causes calluses, which then put more pressure on the area. Eventually, unnoticed, a neuropathic ulcer may form beneath the calluses, becoming infected and leading to serious trouble if it is unchecked.

See Chapter 13 for advice on avoiding this kind of foot problem before it starts. Once an ulcer develops, it must be treated immediately and vigorously if you don't want to be in for a long siege. The infection must be drained and a course of antibiotics begun *promptly*. Then the pressure must be relieved, either by staying off your feet or by special wedges or inner soles in your shoes.

Because of the potential seriousness of an ulcer, your feet should be examined constantly by you and periodically by both your doctor and your podiatrist.

## THE RARER NEUROPATHIES

A few other neuropathic effects include:

• Orthostatic hypotension, which is temporary low pressure occurring when you stand or sit up suddenly or raise your head. This makes you lightheaded, dizzy, and sometimes unsteady on your feet for a few moments. Medication such as Midodrine can help, along with support panty hose to help constrict the blood vessels in the legs.

• Abnormal sweating may be a form of neuropathy, especially when it appears on the face (or *half* the face) after eating.

• "Dry foot," when the feet don't produce sweat and so tend to dry out and crack. Or the opposite, feet that are particularly sweaty.

• Radicular pain, a sharp abdominal pain, which usually recedes after a while.

• Charcot's foot, a phenomenon that is frequently triggered by neuropathy. It usually starts with painless fractures of the bones of the foot and progresses if untreated to muscle atrophy and joint damage until the foot becomes deformed. Treatment is to catch the problem early, stay off your feet, and wear special footwear.

• Sexual impotence after many years of diabetes, and retrograde ejaculation, which means the semen flows back into the bladder rather than out of the penis (see Chapter 15).

## WHAT'S THE OUTLOOK FOR NEUROPATHY?

Because not much is known about what actually causes neuropathy, not much is known about what to do about it either. In some cases, medication can be helpful. In others, the symptoms disappear as mysteriously as they came, and most usually go away eventually or markedly improve.

In the early stages, 100 mgs of vitamin $B_1$ taken daily can be effective. If it isn't, try $B_{12}$ injections up to 20 units. If you wish you can inject this along with your insulin. A daily dose of 1,000 I.U. of vitamin E may help alleviate the discomfort.

Experimental work is now under way to test the effectiveness of a drug called myonisotol in increasing nerve conduction. This is a substance found in the nerve coverings, and also in cantaloupes and peanuts. On the chance this natural form may help you, test it out by eating a quarter of a cantaloupe in place of other vitamin C fruits in the morning.

If your neuropathy causes pain, you and your doctor will have to come up with medication that works for you, taking care that, in your eagerness to dull the discomfort, you don't become dependent on the drugs. This can become more of a problem than the discomfort.

Unfortunately, no medication eases the pain for everyone so you may have to keep trying one after the other. Sharp pains may respond to carbamazepine (Tegretol). Some people are helped by calcitonin nasal spray, a source of calcium, or Clonidine, a blood-pressure medication. Others find relief by applying capsaicin (Zostrex) to the skin two to four times a day. If you use capsaicin, keep your hands away from your eyes after you use it—it's made of red pepper and it stings.

A study of the effectiveness of nerve growth factor (NGF) as a treatment for neuropathy is currently under way at the Albert Einstein College of Medicine and, so far, the prospects seem good. A drug called Tolrestat, used in Mexico, Ireland, and Italy but not yet in the United States, seems to improve autonomic function. Mexiletene, a medication under investigation in Sweden, is reported to alleviate the severe pain sometimes associated with neuropathy. A procedure called electrical spinal cord stimulation (ESCS) has been found in tests to help some people whose symptoms do not respond to other treatments. And there is testimonial evidence that evening primrose oil, found in health food stores, may provide relief.

Meanwhile, exercise regularly, don't smoke, limit alcohol to only a few drinks a week, and inspect your feet and legs daily. And let's not forget *control*. Obviously, good control over your blood-sugar level may help you avoid the neuropathies in the first place. And it is quite possible it can prevent further progress of problems you already have.

NOTE: if you have been in poor control for a long time, have developed neuropathy, but now seek tight control, you may find that any neuropathic discomforts are aggravated at first. This may tempt you to revert to your old bad habits. But hold on. If you stay with it, you will soon feel better.

## DIABETES AND YOUR TEETH

No doubt you'd like to keep a complete set of your very own teeth forever—nobody looks forward to dropping his teeth into a glass every night. If so, you are going to have to take extraordinarily good care of them, because you are more susceptible than most people to gum disease, the major cause of tooth loss. That is another result of the effect of diabetes on the body's myriad tiny capillaries. The thickened walls of the little blood vessels make oxygen-vs.-waste exchange less efficient. And you are then more likely to develop infections that are difficult to get rid of. If your diabetes is poorly controlled, your white blood cells, whose job it is to fight off bacteria, are less effective in their battle against infection, causing an infection to become more severe and harder to heal. The reason is that the white cells don't migrate as quickly as they should to the source of the infection and, once there, are not as vigorous in their battle against the offending bacteria.

## BRUSHING AND FLOSSING

What this means is that you must practice excellent dental hygiene so you won't run into these problems. Using a soft toothbrush (hard ones can scratch the gums) and a fluoride toothpaste, brush your teeth carefully after every meal. Don't scrub, but use light downward strokes.

Then *every night* before going to bed and just after you have brushed your teeth, take some unwaxed dental floss and floss out the plaque that accumulates around each tooth under the gumline in places that the toothbrush doesn't reach. Gently, gently! Ask your dentist or dental hygienist to give you a lesson in the proper way to do this: Wind the ends of the floss around your two forefingers, then *gently* work the taut center section between two teeth. Do not snap it in because you must be careful not to injure your gums. Then, first to the left, then to the right, curving the floss into a U-shape, gently dislodge the plaque from around the gumline of each tooth. When you have done this between all your teeth, rinse out your mouth.

If you are not sure you have done a good job with the flossing, you can buy some special vegetable dye that will show you the places you have missed. It is made for this purpose.

Gum massage is another useful preventive measure because it improves the circulation. After each brushing, take your fingers and gently but firmly give your gums a good rub. Better yet, use a special gum massager with a rubber tip. And check out your dentist's opinion of a water-jet gadget that is designed to get rid of the debris caught in and around your teeth that isn't dislodged by brushing.

See your dentist *at least* every four to six months, both for a good cleaning—it's important that hardened plaque or tartar is removed that often—and to check out your gums. Go to the dentist within the week if you notice any sign of trouble—swelling, soreness, sensitivity, dark spots, white or red patches—anywhere in your mouth. If you have developed periodontal disease, immediate treatment is what you need. Be sure your dentist is thoroughly knowledgeable about gum disease, diabetes, and current methods of treatment and, if necessary, sends you to a periodontist, a dentist who specializes in gum disease.

## MORE TOOTH TIPS

• Before you have any dental work done, *including cleaning,* which frequently results in injured gums, you should be "covered" by antibiotics. That means, because you are susceptible to infections, all preventive measures should be taken automatically. You should have three days of antibiotic treatment—the day before, the day of, and the day after the dental work.

• Keep in mind that some drugs, such as Dilantin, can have an adverse effect on your gums.

• If you have periodontal work done on your gums, that doesn't mean you can now forget the flossing and the massage. The problems will return if you don't work hard to prevent them.

• Be sure to get your diabetes under excellent control *before* having any periodontal surgery, so you will have the best chance of fast healing.

• If, because of periodontal work or extractions, you must eat soft or liquid foods for a while, remember that you must still abide by a proper diabetic diet. Liquids are fine, but they do contain calories and perhaps sugar and must be accounted for just as if they were solid foods. If you are confused about substitutions (see Chapter 4), work it out with your doctor or a dietitian *before* you get into trouble.

## DIABETES AND YOUR SKIN

For all the same reasons that you tend to get infections more easily than people with normal blood sugar, and have a harder time fighting them off, you may discover you have skin problems more often too. If you do, look to your control. Though the blame for these may be shared by microvascular changes and sluggish white cells that aren't so quick to attack bacteria and other invaders, remember that high sugar is the real villain, and that skin infections are often the direct result of poorly controlled diabetes. In fact, boils, styes, inflammation around the nails, and other eruptions are often the clue that makes a physician suspect diabetes in the first place. Poor control also causes dry, itchy skin, which you may scratch and irritate, issuing an invitation to an invasion of bacteria.

Poor control promotes the appearance of fungus or yeast infections of the vagina in women, of the groin in men, and sometimes of the anus regardless of your gender. Your doctor can prescribe effective medication. Your job is to use it faithfully and get yourself back in good condition. Fungi also make homes in armpits, between fingers and toes, around the nails, and in other moist places. A drug called Lamisil, taken topically or orally, is very effective against fungal infections such as athlete's foot of the feet and hands.

## SPOTS AND OTHER PROBLEMS

Fairly common among long-term diabetics is spotted leg syndrome or skin spots. These little brown pockmarks that start out looking like reddish bruises usually appear on the shins where tiny end capillaries have shut down. They don't hurt and they don't get worse, though we know of no way to get rid of them.

A skin condition, necrobiosis lipoidica diabeticorum (NLD), is the special province of diabetics and it, too, is worrisome chiefly for cosmetic reasons. Necrobiosis is the appearance, frequently on the lower legs, of patches of reddish-brown lesions. These become areas of tight, shiny skin like glazed parchment paper that is indented because of a loss of subcutaneous fat just beneath it. Sometimes they are itchy or even painful; or they may crack. The spots are often discolored, but they tend to fade with time, although this may take a few years. Some doctors have successfully treated NLD with fine-needle injections of cortisone, though usually no treatment is needed except to prevent injury or infection.

Ulcers, which start out as a skin problem, soon become more than that if the infection deepens and extends into the surrounding tissue. If you discover even the smallest indication of infection, especially on your legs or feet, call your doctor immediately. Prompt treatment to avert big trouble is what you need.


## INSULIN ATROPHY AND HYPERTROPHY

A cosmetic problem called lipodystrophy (insulin atrophy and hypertrophy) is, happily, becoming much less common among diabetics today as purer insulins are developed. Insulin atrophy, which appears in areas where insulin injections are given frequently, is a loss of fatty tissue just below the skin, causing large depressions that look scooped out. This can make a person—and usually this happens to young women—most unhappy, although usually the areas eventually fill in again and disappear.

Sometimes insulin injections promote an abnormal buildup of fat, and so you have lumps instead of hollows, or occasionally both. This is called insulin hypertrophy.

To prevent hypertrophy, don't inject into identical sites continually. Rotate your shots so you don't hit the same place more than once a month. Keep a record of your sites to help you do this.

Diabetic blisters (bullosa diabeticorum) are painless raised areas that look like burn blisters. These are quite rare and happen to people whose diabetes is out of control. To get rid of them, attend to your blood sugar. They will disappear in a few weeks.

Small, hard pealike bumps with red halos and an itch are another sign of lack of diabetic control and will disappear when you are in better shape. This condition is known as eruptive xanthomatosis.

## EVERYDAY SKIN CARE

If you allow your skin to become dry and chapped—and dry skin is a characteristic of diabetics (in fact, the skin becomes dehydrated when your control is poor)—you will not only be inviting bacteria, but you will lower the skin's ability to serve as a barrier to the loss of body water. Don't take too many baths, especially in cold weather. Don't wash too often with soap, and avoid disinfectants or solvents. Try super-fatted soaps. Wear gloves and scarves and warm socks or stockings when you're out in the cold.

To add moisture to your skin and protect it, soak (your whole body or just the dry area) in warm water for several minutes, pat off the excess water, then apply a greasy ointment like petroleum jelly or lanolin, or a good dry-skin cream or lotion.

If you use bath oil, pour the oil in the tub *after* you have soaked yourself for a while. In this way, your skin will first absorb some water which the oil will help to retain. If you put the oil in the water before you have absorbed some moisture into your skin, it will form a barrier to that moisture.

The same principle applies to moisturizing lotion or cream whose purpose is to seal water in. Wet your skin and pat it almost dry before applying the moisturizer.

# *12*

# RULES FOR SICK DAYS

Just like everybody else, you are going to get sick occasionally. But, unlike everybody else, you will discover your life promptly becomes much more complicated simply because you are a diabetic with an infection. Infections can be more difficult to get rid of and often more severe for you because your defenses may not be the best. Besides, with most illnesses your insulin requirements will rise, sometimes quite dramatically.

All this means that control may be hard to maintain during an illness, so now your objective is not only to recover from the illness but also to avoid acidosis and a trip to the hospital.

If you are on diet alone or diet plus oral agents, remember you are not immune to high blood sugars, acetone, and acidosis when you are sick. You may need temporary shots of insulin to get through, so never neglect your blood tests. Instead of one a day, increase them to three or four. If you normally take insulin, your chief occupation now will be testing your blood and adjusting your dose according to your doctor's instructions. You will undoubtedly need more insulin, maybe two or three times more than usual.

When you are sick, you must live strictly by the rules:

RULE 1:   Stay in close touch with your doctor. The doctor is the person who must make the medical decisions, some major, some minor, when you are sick. Remember the telephone is your friend. If you see a problem evolving during the day, however, call early. Any doctor would rather hear from you at 6 or 10 P.M. than 2 A.M., but better 2 A.M. than not at all if you are in bad shape.

If you feel your physician doesn't like to be bothered by frequent (not excessive) phone calls or is not providing the guidance you need, find another one. Check with the American Diabetes Association or Juvenile Diabetes Foundation in your area for a recommendation.

RULE 2:   When you are sick, *check your blood at least four times a day,* before each meal and at bedtime. If you are seriously ill, check it every *two* hours. Just as you are never too tired to breathe, you are *never* too tired or sick or weak to test yourself. You must know where your blood sugar stands because the test will tell you what to do next.

RULE 3:   When blood sugar is high, the diabetic who takes insulin must compensate with extra insulin, the fast-acting (Regular) variety. Your doctor will tell you how much to take. It may be 5 units every two hours if your sugar is more than 250, or, if that doesn't do the job, 10 or more units every two hours.

When you get a high sugar reading, *always test for acetone.* The presence of acetone *along with* high sugar means you need extra insulin quickly. Now you may require even *more* extra Regular insulin every two hours until the sugar comes down, according to your doctor's instructions. This is vital if you are going to avoid acidosis.

After you have lowered your blood sugar with increased insulin, it would be wise to set your alarm clock for 3 A.M. Check your blood sugar and eat something if it is low.

*However, if your sugar is normal and your acetone is positive,* take only your usual dose of insulin. If your sugar is low—under 100 mgs—skip the Regular insulin and take your usual dose of Intermediate. In this case, high acetone means the acetone has not been entirely washed out of the body (it may remain for about 24 hours after your sugar has been regulated back to normal); or that your body lacks its primary fuel—sugar—and is burning fat, one of the end products of which is acetone. You now need carbohydrate—juice, bread, cereal, milk, etc.—plus some protein to avoid an insulin reaction now and later in the day and to give your body its normal fuel. Check with your doctor.

Sickness is rarely a major diabetic problem for a person controlled only by diet, but it can be. Even you can develop acidosis if you allow high sugars to persist without taking action. Call your doctor if you have high sugars for more than 24 hours. You may require temporary insulin because the stress of illness can raise your insulin requirement far beyond the ability of your pancreas to produce it.

When you take oral agents, your insulin needs will rise during an infection because of the additional release of glucose from the liver. The result may be that the amount of insulin produced by your own pancreas with the help of the oral agent won't be enough to cover the sugar and prevent the end result of acidosis. Your doctor must make the decision as to whether you should take more of the oral agent until your blood sugar drops, or whether you will need insulin injections temporarily. When you have reached or come close to your maximum dosage of oral hypoglycemic agents, your physician may add a different kind of oral agent such as Glucophage, or Precose. But if you continue to have high sugar and produce acetone, you will be instructed to use insulin—either alone or as a supplement to the pills—until your glucose levels are normal once more. Call your doctor, who will probably prescribe five to ten units of quick-acting insulin every two hours.

RULE 4: Always keep Regular insulin on hand, whether or not you normally use it. This fast-acting insulin is what you may need to counteract high sugar quickly.

RULE 5: *Never* omit your daily insulin, *even if you are eating less than usual or not at all,* although you may need a smaller dose. Your diabetes does not disappear just because you can't eat, and your liver continues to manufacture glucose, perhaps much more than usual.

If your blood tests are *normal* or *high,* take your usual dose. Then consult with your doctor about an extra amount.

If your sugar is *low* but you cannot eat, take *half* your usual dose. But *never* take nothing or you will end up with acidosis.

Continue to test throughout the day. Don't wait till tomorrow, hoping you'll wake up cured. You may wake up in the hospital instead.

If you are on oral agents, you can omit your pills when you cannot eat much and your blood sugar is below 100 mgs. Always, of course, check with your doctor.

RULE 6: Try to eat. Even if you are not hungry or you are nauseated, you can usually find something that will go down and stay there. To prevent acidosis, you need at least 50 to 60 grams of carbohydrate a day. If you can't stick to your usual diet plan, switch over to food that goes down most easily and eat it in smaller amounts spaced throughout the day. If you can't eat normal meals, now is the time for you to eat carbohydrates, so that you get sufficient fuel.

Try toast, crackers, soups, a small amount of regular ginger ale, yogurt, juices, custard, ice cream. Perhaps grapefruit, eggnog, cereal. Your goal should be 10 grams of carbohydrate an hour.

If liquids are all you can manage, drink your food, remembering that you must have sufficient carbohydrate as well as salt to replace the salt lost by excessive urination. Clear soup, salty broth, tea with sugar, juice, milk, regular (not diet) ginger ale or cola to give you the carbohydrate you need may appeal to you. Take some about every half hour in small amounts.

If you can't eat or drink at all, inform your doctor *immediately.* If you can't reach your doctor, go to an emergency room before you're in really big trouble.

### Easy-to-Eat Foods

| | |
|---|---|
| Applesauce | Jams or jellies, regular |
| Bread | Jell-O, regular |
| Broth, bouillon | Popsicle |
| Cereal | Postum |
| Coffee | Sherbet |
| Cottage cheese | Soft drinks, regular |
| Crackers | Soups |
| Custard | Sugar |
| Egg | Tapioca |
| Eggnog | Tea |
| Fruit juices | Tomato juice |
| Ice cream | Vegetable cocktail |
| Ice milk | Yogurt |

RULE 7: Try to control vomiting as quickly as possible. Three ounces of regular ginger ale or cola every hour often acts as an antiemetic and provides the needed carbohydrate too. If that doesn't banish the nausea, your doctor can prescribe a suppository or give you an antinausea injection. Tigan suppositories (200 mgs for adults or 100 mgs for children who weigh less than 30 pounds) every eight hours, or Compazine suppositories (up to 25 mgs for adults, 5 mgs for older children, 2.5 mgs for young children) every eight hours are usually effective.

If you can't eat or drink at all or you are continuing to vomit, call your doctor *immediately.* You may need intravenous infusions of saline solution and/or glucose.

Continue to take your usual insulin or oral agent, plus Regular insulin every two hours if your sugar is high.

RULE 8: Control diarrhea as quickly as possible, too, because it can cause the loss of valuable fluids and carbohydrates. Usually a drug such as Lomotil works well, but if you have diarrhea and nausea at the same time, you won't be able to keep it down nor can you use suppositories. An intramuscular injection of Compazine, which your doctor can prescribe, may be the solution. *Call the doctor* for instructions.

RULE 9:   There is no need to stay in bed, but it's important to rest as much as possible. Do not exercise. If you are very sick, it would be advisable to have someone to take care of you.

RULE 10:   If you are taking antibiotics, you will have an increased tendency to get fungal infections—vaginitis, rectal itching, skin infections. When you are given an antibiotic, you should also be given lactobacillus, perhaps acidophilis tablets. Plain yogurt eaten in place of fruit or bread may help prevent an overgrowth of the fungi. Always check the container to make sure it has live cultures.

RULE 11:   Check all medications for sugar. Many cold medicines as well as other drugs are loaded with it and can throw your control off in a hurry. Sudafed and Triaminic syrups, for example, contain 3½ grams of carbohydrate per teaspoon. If you take three teaspoons a day for a cold, you are adding 10½ grams of unwanted simple sugar to your bloodstream. Robitussin cough syrup contains 2.8 grams per teaspoon, or 11.2 extra grams when you take the recommended 4 teaspoons a day. Other cold medicines have similar carbohydrate contents.

   You certainly should not add this much sugar to your body at a time when you are already under the stress of infection and your glucose tolerance is disturbed because of the release of cortisone from your adrenal glands. It is possible, however, to get medications without sugar. Cough medicines that at this writing are sugar-free include Cerose-DM, Contact Jr. Liquid, Naldecon Senior DX Syrup, Naldecon Senior EX Syrup, Polyhistine DM, Scot-Tussin DM Liquid, and Scot-Tussin Syrup.

RULE 12:   *Keep a careful record* of all your test results, insulin intake, food, and drink. Omit nothing. Write this information down so that you can refer to it when you discuss your situation with your doctor. Include comments on how you feel, whether you are vomiting, have diarrhea, a temperature, etc., each time you record your test results.

## INJURIES AND SURGERY

Both surgery and physical injuries are an assault on your diabetic control because they stimulate the body's defense mechanism to pour out cortisone and adrenaline which increase your blood sugar. So you must double your efforts at these times to maintain good control, making frequent tests and perhaps taking additional insulin.

If you are in good control, you'll have no special problems recovering from surgery and will heal just about as quickly as anyone else. When you expect surgery, bring your sugar into the normal range and keep it there, if you can. Otherwise, you may find that acidosis lurks just around the corner and that you'll heal with difficulty. The best-known anabolic (tissue-building) agent is insulin.

Of course, your doctor is in charge when you are in the hospital and will make adjustments in your medication to regulate your sugar both during the operative procedure and postoperatively. Your insulin will be increased, or, if you don't normally take it, you may have to go the insulin route temporarily until you are stable once more.

When surgery is scheduled, ask your doctor to make you the first case of the day so your normal routine will be disturbed as little as possible. If you are on an oral agent, you don't want to take that morning's dose because you won't be eating before the operation and your sugar may fall very low. If you are on insulin, you will probably be given an intravenous glucose infusion and half of your insulin dose on the morning of the surgery, then insulin as needed after the surgery. I strongly advise that you arrange to be in the care of a qualified diabetologist in addition to the surgeon at this time.

Even when you are in the hospital, the rules still apply. "They gave it to me" is no excuse for eating so much carbohydrate that your blood sugar will go sky-high. If you are suffering from an infection or the stress of surgery, your blood sugar will tend to run high anyway—don't make it worse by eating the wrong foods (see Chapter 4).

## BEWARE DRUG INTERACTIONS

If you have an illness that requires you take a drug, be sure your doctor remembers you are a diabetic. If you go to a specialist who does not know your history, give out the information immediately. Not only does your diabetes affect your illness, but the drugs prescribed may affect your diabetes.

For example, oral cortisone raises insulin requirements. Diabetics on insulin may need a higher dose, and those on diet or oral agents may need to take insulin while taking cortisone. People often do not know that prednisone, Medrol, and dexamethasone are cortisone drugs.

Dilantin is a major drug used for epilepsy or convulsive disorders. It has the ability to inhibit insulin release, so even people with borderline diabetes can be thrown out of control when they use this drug. Even though it is sometimes prescribed for diabetic neuropathy, it can be dangerous.

Inderal, a drug commonly prescribed for angina, headaches, and hypertension, can mask an insulin reaction as mentioned in Chapter 9. When blood sugar is low, the adrenal glands secrete adrenaline which releases sugar from the liver. A rapid heartbeat, sweating, and other symptoms generally alert you to the fact that you are becoming hypoglycemic, but Inderal blocks this effect so that you may not be aware of your precarious situation. Certain other drugs affect the action of the oral agents, too, enhancing their effectiveness and sometimes producing hypoglycemic reactions. To repeat the list, these include: Coumadin, Butazoladine, Benemid, Dilantin, sulfonamides, mood ameliorators, and a number of other medications.

The action of drugs such as barbiturates, sedatives, and hypnotics can be greatly prolonged when they are taken together with oral agents. In addition, the effect of the oral agents may be prolonged as well. Don't take any chances. Before you take a new drug, be sure to check out its effect on your diabetes.

# 13

# WATCHING YOUR FEET

When you are a diabetic, you hear a lot about taking good care of your feet. It may seem like a minor issue, but it's extremely important that you follow all the rules about foot care if you want to avoid some very unpleasant problems in the future. Any injuries or infections of the feet and ankles and even lower legs are potentially very dangerous to the diabetic. They can lead to serious complications that can be treated only by drastic surgery, which you don't even want to think about. The most common reason for the amputation of feet and legs is long-term diabetes, so the big word now is *prevention*. Don't let anything get started. And if it should, go *immediately* to your doctor.

A diabetic, especially if control has been poor for a number of years, tends to have poor circulation in the legs and feet. This is particularly true for older people. The small arteries become narrower and cannot carry the optimum amounts of blood, oxygen, and infection-fighting white cells to these extremities. That makes diabetics particularly susceptible to injuries, calluses, and infections such as carbuncles, boils, and athlete's foot, which can become serious problems *very* quickly. It also tends to reduce sweat production which can lead to dry skin that cracks and becomes infected more easily.

Sometimes the nerve endings, as well as the circulation, are affected. Diabetics often have neuropathy—damage to the small sensory nerves—and that means you may not have the feeling in your feet that you once had. You can cut yourself, wear shoes that rub, step on sharp objects, or burn yourself and never realize it. You can get athlete's foot or other infections without knowing it. Meanwhile, the wound or infection can rapidly turn into a major problem. For a nondiabetic a little cut, a rub, a blister, a fungus may be only an annoyance. For a diabetic, any foot injury that's neglected can lead to an ulcer. This could be the start of deep trouble, so you can't let it go, even for a few days.

That's why, though you may find it a nuisance, you must consciously pay attention to your feet every single day. Actually it's easy and takes only a few minutes, and it wouldn't be a bad idea if everyone did the same thing. Feet are rarely anyone's favorite part of the body and are usually totally ignored and maltreated until they start causing some discomfort. But you can't afford to ignore yours—you *must* head off any problems before they begin if you possibly can.

You have to abide by a list of simple rules of hygiene, remember a number of things you should and should not do, make periodic appointments with a reputable podiatrist, and, most important, waste no time in checking with your podiatrist and/or your doctor if you notice the slightest sign of a problem, even a small discoloration. Never assume that whatever it is will just clear up on its own. It might, but it might not. Never treat your feet yourself except under the direction of your doctor. Never assume anything is too minor to worry about. Always remember *you must not wait* until you feel pain to become concerned—you may not feel a thing and yet be brewing serious problems. Don't take any chances.

## BE SURE YOU GET A THOROUGH EXAMINATION

Whenever you see your doctor, whether for a routine exam or because something seems amiss, insist on a close inspection of your feet and legs. You should remove your shoes and socks so the doctor can check the pulses of your feet and the integrity of your skin, look for calluses and corns and other problems, compare one foot against the other, and screen you for neuropathy.

All of these procedures are essential if you are going to avoid serious foot problems. To test for a dangerous decline in sensation that can signal nerve damage and lead to neuropathic ulcers, the doctor may use a simple inexpensive monofilament device, a special brush with a single nylon bristle. The brush is pressed against various spots on the feet and lower legs to gauge the feeling in these areas. It has been estimated that annual testing for lost sensation could prevent 80 to 90 percent of all foot amputations caused by these problems.

In addition, the physician should check the blood flow in your feet and legs with a Doppler meter because you also have a tendency to have compromised blood circulation in your lower extremities that can lead to serious complications.

If you have an ulcer, you will require an X ray and/or a white-blood-cell scan to look for bone damage or joint degeneration and tests to rule out infection.

## EVERYDAY FOOT CARE

### Washing

Wash your feet every day. Yes, every day. They must be kept clean. This does not mean soaking them, not a wise practice for diabetics. In fact, it is dangerous and actually encourages infection by softening the skin so much that it may break easily and provide a home for bacteria and fungi.

Because your skin is probably very dry, use a nonalkaline soap. (If you're not sure which brands are nonalkaline, ask your druggist for one. It will not require a prescription.) Be especially careful to avoid deodorant soaps, which are particularly drying.

Be sure the water is only warm (below 92° F.), *never* hot.

*Danger!* If you have a loss of pain perception, common in many diabetics, you may not notice the water is too hot if you carelessly dip your feet in without testing it first. Don't test with your toe. Use your hand or your elbow. Or use a thermometer. One thing you must not have is burned feet.

Now take a soft towel and carefully dry your feet. Do not rub between your toes, because the skin here is thin and delicate, but pat off the moisture to avoid irritation.

## Examining

This is the moment to take a close look at every square millimeter of your feet and lower legs. Every day. If your eyesight isn't good or you have trouble bending over that far, enlist someone else to do this. We'll say it again: If you see any broken skin, peeling, redness, irritation, blisters, bruises, swelling, *anything* that even vaguely strikes you as unusual, don't treat it yourself and don't waste a moment. Go immediately to your podiatrist or physician.

By the way, every diabetic should have a good podiatrist, a specialist in foot care. Podiatrists are frequently much more knowledgeable about foot and leg problems than most physicians.

## SKIN CARE

After you have examined your feet closely, sprinkle some baby powder between your toes. Then gently rub a skin-softening lotion or cream on your feet and legs to counteract the dryness, except between your toes where you do not want moisture. Avoid any lotions that contain medication or alcohol.

## PEDICURES

For most diabetics, it is an excellent idea to go to a podiatrist as often as necessary to have your toenails trimmed. It is much better than doing it yourself. That's because a small slip of the scissors can be the start of trouble. Especially if your toenails are thick—as they often are in older people—it is best for an expert to do the job. Besides, your visit will be an opportunity for this expert to check out your feet to be sure all is well. You will have a chance to ask questions and get advice, eliminating vague worries from your mind and forestalling any ill-advised self-treatment.

If you are going to do the pedicuring yourself at any time, keep the following rules in mind. Use manicuring scissors with blunt rounded tips, the kind used for cutting babies' nails. Cut your nails after a bath so they will be soft. Trim them *straight across,* even with the ends of your toes. If they are too long, you will have pressure on the nail bed; if they are too short, they will not protect your toes as they are intended to do and may expose the fragile skin beneath them.

Never cut cuticles or skin. Don't cut in at the corners, because you will not only be in danger of cutting into the skin but you will also invite ingrown toenails. Don't use a nail file to keep your toenails in shape because you may unwittingly file your skin and irritate it. But you should use an emery board with a light touch to smooth down any rough edges.

If someone else does this job for you, be sure that person knows how to do it the right way. Give him/her this chapter to read.

## EVEN MORE ADVICE

Now you may be thinking that all these rules about your feet are excessive, but we are going to add more anyway. If you want to stay in good shape, with two strong healthy feet holding you up for the rest of your life, don't skip to the next chapter but keep reading.

## CHECK OUT YOUR FOOTWEAR

Change your socks every day, more often if they get wet or your feet sweat a lot. If they don't fit perfectly, give them away. Your socks must not be too large or too small. They must not form wrinkles in your shoes. They must not have seams. They must not have holes. They must not be mended. Stretch socks or hosiery are not a good idea for you because they may restrict circulation or put pressure on your toes. Never wear socks or stockings with elasticized tops for the same reason. Furthermore, garters are out. Cotton or wool socks are the best choices because they are more absorbent than the synthetic fibers. When hiking, wear lightweight socks under regular-weight socks.

Never, never wear shoes that don't fit perfectly and comfortably. Each foot has 26 bones and 78 joints that must be well treated. Be sure there is enough room to accommodate all your toes in their natural positions, and that the heel is snug enough not to slide up and down. Buy shoes in the afternoon when your feet are the largest, and always have your feet measured standing, not sitting. Feet tend to get larger as you get older, so do not assume you wear the same size without checking. Choose shoes made of leather, not plastic, to allow more air circulation. If you are an animal rights supporter who won't wear leather, find fabric shoes or plastic shoes with pores or airholes.

If your sensory perception is not too good, you may not feel rubbing, so be sure to watch for it every time you take off your shoes and during your daily ablutions. Don't wear open toes—closed toes give much more protection. Break in new shoes gradually by wearing them around the house and then on short jaunts.

Get in the habit of feeling the insides of your shoes before you put them on, to be sure there aren't any protruding nails, bumps, torn linings, or rough spots that may be hazards.

If you can't find shoes that fit right, consult with your podiatrist who may have a solution for you.

Going barefoot, even in the house, is not for diabetics. The minute you step out of bed in the morning, put on a pair of slippers or shoes. Wear swim shoes or sneakers on the beach. Don't take a chance on stubbing your toe, getting a splinter, stepping on a piece of glass or a sharp shell, burning your feet on hot sand or cement.

## SOME MORE IMPORTANT DON'TS

• Don't use medications or chemicals on your feet unless prescribed by your doctor (and be sure the doctor remembers you are diabetic). This includes over-the-counter foot remedies. Powerful medications, such as iodine, or medicated materials such as corn plasters, can destroy tissue or cause burns to delicate skin. A good rule is: If you can't put it on your face, don't put it on your feet. Tinted medicines, mercurochrome, for example, are taboo too because they can camouflage inflammation.

• Don't try bathroom surgery with scissors, razors, or even pumice stones or corn pads. If you develop a corn or a callus—which you shouldn't because you've thrown out your ill-fitting shoes—leave it alone! Let your podiatrist treat it. If you have poor weight distribution, which may be causing the corns or calluses, this specialist may make a special mold for you to wear in your shoe to correct the problem. Do not mess with blisters either. Never open them.

• Don't use heat on your feet. Never put your feet in hot water. Remember to test the bath water with your hand or elbow. Stay out of saunas, steam rooms, whirlpool baths—most of them are too hot for your feet. Apply lots of sunscreen lotion when you are out in the sun—don't let your feet get sunburned. *Never* use hot-water bottles or heating pads.

• Don't let your feet get too chilled, either. Because your blood vessels are probably narrower and more constricted when you have diabetes, it's easier for you to get frostbite. Invest in warm (but smooth) socks and roomy boots for cold weather. But don't wear boots indoors all day, because they can impede your circulation and, because they are warm, make your feet sweat and become susceptible to bacteria.

• Don't use adhesive tape. It can irritate the skin or even pull some skin away when you take it off. Instead, use "ouchless" bandages or MMM tape.

• Don't stay in bed for more than a day without protecting your heels with an "egg-crate" pad under your feet and special heel pads to shield them from rubbing. This is especially important when you are hospitalized because ulcers can develop very quickly on diabetic feet. Insist on these protections *on Day One* of your stay. Do not wait for a problem to develop before taking action.

• Don't smoke. Just one cigarette will constrict your peripheral blood vessels to an astonishing degree. Since yours are probably already narrower than normal, smoking will only compound the situation.

That is a lot of nevers and don'ts, but all must be heeded.

## GOT A PROBLEM?

Do not waste a second if you notice a lesion on a foot or a leg. Get yourself to your doctor that very day because lesions must be treated aggressively and quickly with oral or topical antibiotics if they are not to become serious problems. If your physician is not experienced in dealing with diabetic ulcers, ask for a referral.

## GET ENOUGH EXERCISE

You need some kind of exercise every day because it will improve your circulation and encourage collateral vascular development. When your feet and the rest of you are in good condition, there is no exercise you can't do—from tennis to running to ice hockey. Nonathletes can move their blood around most efficiently by swimming or walking briskly at least a half hour every day.

Caution: if you have a foot or lower leg injury or infection, this is not the time for exercise. Even if it doesn't hurt, walking on injuries can damage them further.

# 14

# PREGNANCY PROBLEMS

Can I have a baby? Will I have problems conceiving? Will the baby be normal? How risky is pregnancy for me? How will it affect my diabetes? Will the baby be diabetic? These are questions of immense importance to young women with diabetes. Happily, the answers today are astonishingly positive. Not many years ago, a diabetic woman conceived with difficulty and embarked on a hazardous trip when she became pregnant, with a good chance of losing her baby on the way and endangering her own health.

But today, the vast majority of diabetic women can have healthy babies, with only a slightly higher than normal statistical chance of miscarriage, congenital anomalies, and stillbirths, even in the presence of some serious diabetic complications. According to the Joslin Clinic, the fetal survival rate of diabetic pregnancies is now about 97 percent, while the rate for nondiabetics is 98 or 99 percent. That is a remarkably small difference. And maternal deaths today are almost nonexistent.

Managing a diabetic pregnancy, however, requires excellent medical care, as well as complete cooperation on your part. This venture demands total dedication and motivation, hard work, time, and attention. Besides, a diabetic pregnancy can be expensive. You may need the expert medical care of a whole team of specialists, many office visits, perhaps a number of hospitalizations, sophisticated laboratory tests, possibly a cesarean delivery.

For a happy outcome to a diabetic pregnancy, extremely tight blood-sugar control is the key. What we look for is blood sugar under 100 mgs percent before breakfast and less than 120 mg two hours after eating. This is not so easy for an insulin-dependent woman, though it can definitely be achieved if you work at it. If you are controlled by diet alone, it is all much simpler. You may get along well simply by watching what you eat, paying strict attention to your sugar levels, and staying in close touch with your obstetrician and internist. Or you may need insulin temporarily because you don't produce enough yourself to satisfy the huge demands of a pregnancy.

If you are normally controlled by diet and oral hypoglycemic agents, you must now switch to insulin until after the baby is born. This is because the oral agents will not only stimulate your pancreas but the baby's as well. Because it is not yet known whether the oral drugs cross over into breast milk, it is also recommended—if you are going to breastfeed—that you continue on insulin until the baby is weaned if strict diet does not give you sufficient control.

## PLAN AHEAD

Ideally, you should have your babies early in life. And you should plan ahead, decide when to conceive, get yourself in the best possible physical shape before you begin your pregnancy, because the first few weeks of life are the times when your baby's organs are formed. This means your diabetes is under excellent control, you are not overweight, and you have resolved any important medical problems before you start off. Some doctors even recommend, as a prelude to pregnancy, that a diabetic woman check into the hospital for at least a few days for evaluation and glucose regulation. If you followed the earlier rules this should not be necessary. At least one study has demonstrated that the babies of women with the lowest hemoglobin A1c, blood-sugar levels measured over two or three months, have the fewest abnormalities.

Once you are pregnant, don't waste a moment starting your prenatal care. Your insulin requirements will change radically and quickly. Good diabetic control—whether or not you take insulin—is particularly important during the first two months, the time when much of the baby's initial development occurs.

A team of medical experts will manage your pregnancy—an obstetrician, a diabetologist (a physician who is a diabetic specialist), perhaps a dietitian, laboratory technicians, later a pediatrician who specializes in perinatology. You will probably visit the obstetrician every week or two until about the thirtieth week, then more often after that. You may consult with the dietitian now and then and see your diabetic specialist twice a month. There are also high-risk obstetricians and neonatologists who specialize in diabetic pregnancies.

## CONCEIVING YOUR BABY

If you are healthy, you can get pregnant just as easily as anyone else. Diabetes does not interfere with your fertility when you are well controlled. A diabetic husband, however, may be a source of conception difficulties (see Chapter 15).

## IF YOUR HUSBAND IS DIABETIC

Having a diabetic husband will not affect your pregnancy at all, whether or not you are diabetic yourself.

## CHOOSING YOUR OBSTETRICIAN

Unfortunately, many good obstetricians do not have expert knowledge of the special problems of diabetic pregnancies.

Nor do many hospitals have the facilities and laboratories you may need. Especially if you take insulin, it is essential that you check out the obstetricians and hospitals in your area. Much depends on the kind of medical care you will receive.

If you are already seeing a diabetologist, this doctor will know where to refer you. If you are not going to a diabetologist, we suggest you find one now, or at least an internist who has been recommended by your local Juvenile Diabetes Foundation or American Diabetes Association affiliate. You will need the services of this doctor along with those of the obstetrician. He/she must be available to you night and day—as this person should be even when you aren't pregnant.

The diabetic organizations will also recommend obstetricians, as well as the best hospital for you. Or you can call the department of obstetrics and gynecology at the nearest large hospital or medical school for the names of doctors with special expertise in diabetic pregnancies. Do not, unless you have no choice and no chance of moving, pick an obstetrician simply because your next-door neighbor likes him. You require a person who is an expert.

## WHAT KIND OF DIABETIC ARE YOU?

Pregnant diabetic women have been classified into eight groups, so potential problems may be more easily predicted. The classifications, originated by Dr. Priscilla White of the Joslin Clinic, range from those with the mildest diabetic indications to those with the most serious complications. Obviously, women who fit in the early categories usually have the fewest difficulties during pregnancy because their diabetes has had less effect on their bodies' ability to go through the incredibly complicated process of creating a baby.

Here are the classes of pregnant diabetic women:

*Class A:* Gestational diabetics, women who have abnormal glucose tolerance during pregnancy only. For them, the condition is transient. They have no symptoms and diet is usually the only treatment they require.

*Class B:* Women whose diabetes began after age twenty and have had it less than ten years. They have no evidence of kidney or eye disease.

*Class C:* Women who have been diabetic for ten to twenty years, and were diagnosed between the ages of ten to nineteen. Again, no evidence of serious complications.

*Class D:* Women who were diagnosed before age 10 and have had diabetes over twenty years. They have early retinopathy and/or some kidney damage, calcified blood vessels of the legs, or hypertension.

*Class R:* Women who have proliferative retinopathy or vitreous hemorrhage.

*Class F:* Women who have developed neuropathy and/or proteinuria over 500 mgs per day.

*Class RF:* Women with arteriosclerotic heart disease.

*Class T:* Women who have had a renal transplantation.

## GESTATIONAL DIABETES

Sometimes women who have never before shown signs of diabetes develop abnormal glucose tolerance for the first time during a pregnancy, especially if they are 20 percent or more over their ideal weight. They are called gestational diabetics, and unless their diabetes preexisted and is only now being discovered, they can expect to lose the disease as soon as the baby is born. Usually they have no overt symptoms and simply require a good diet and sufficient exercise to keep their blood-sugar level normal so that their transient condition won't affect their babies or their deliveries. Occasionally, though, a gestational diabetic will develop very high blood sugar and may need insulin temporarily to bring it down to normal.

It's important to remember that this temporary abnormality is a sign that diabetes may occur sometime later in life and additional pregnancies may add to the strain on an already vulnerable pancreas. Each ten pounds gained after a diabetic pregnancy also increases the risk. And among women who deliver babies weighing over nine pounds at birth, about 25 percent develop the disease within five years, and 60 percent within twelve years.

Untreated, women with gestational diabetes have a high incidence of oversize infants and so an increased incidence of cesarean deliveries. Treated, however, most have normal-size babies.

## WHAT IS A PREDIABETIC?

A prediabetic is someone who is going to become diabetic, and many pregnant women fit into this group. Pregnancy puts a stress on the pancreas, and if your pancreas has inherited a tendency to diabetes, this may be the time when it will become apparent, the more likely the more pregnancies you have. If you are overweight, remember that every 20 percent of excess weight increases your chances even more.

Because pregnancy is such a common time for diabetes to show up, your obstetrician should perform a routine urinalysis at every visit. Sugar in the urine, however, doesn't have to mean you are diabetic. During any pregnancy, the flow of blood to the kidneys increases and sugar absorption decreases, resulting in more spilled sugar than normal.

But increased glucose in the urine must always be investigated. If you are spilling more sugar than normal, your obstetrician will check for sugar in the blood by giving you an isolated glucose tolerance test using 100 grams of sugar. If after one hour you show a blood-glucose level of more than 135 mgs percent, then you will now require a formal glucose tolerance test (see page 26) to confirm a diagnosis of gestational diabetes.

## WHAT IS DIFFERENT ABOUT A DIABETIC PREGNANCY?

Unless you have had diabetes for many years, have serious complications, or are in poor diabetic control, you do not have a higher chance of miscarriage than any other woman. And you will probably carry your baby to term, or close to it. If your diabetes is more severe, your baby may be delivered early.

Because good control is the road to a happy and successful outcome, constant vigilance is essential. Along with all those scheduled visits to your doctors, you must test your blood for sugar four times a day, adjusting your medication accordingly.

Though the insulin you take does not cross the placenta to the fetus, blood sugar does. This means that when your blood sugar goes up, so does the baby's. This stimulates the immature pancreas to produce too much insulin. Excessive insulin promotes the deposition of fat, and so, even if you are a mild diabetic, your baby is likely to be quite large. This fact alone may mean you will need a cesarean delivery. With excellent control, you can probably keep your baby down to a more normal size, however, and have a normal-term delivery.

Severe diabetics, on the other hand, sometimes have very small babies, because vascular complications involving the placenta may restrict the fetal blood supply and therefore the nourishment the fetus receives.

A frequent problem in diabetic pregnancy is hydramnios, an excessive amount of amniotic fluid, which can make you very uncomfortable and perhaps cause premature labor. At the first sign of hydramnios, you will probably be instructed to stay in bed to reduce the volume of fluid.

Other possible special problems include kidney and vascular complications as a result of damage caused by long-term diabetes; and toxemia, a condition that is becoming much less prevalent as knowledge of the value of good control increases. Because in pregnancy there is a greater tendency toward urinary infections, your urine should be checked regularly.

## HOW PREGNANCY AFFECTS YOUR DIABETES

Because carrying a baby is a severe stress on your pancreas, your need for insulin will skyrocket during your pregnancy, doubling or even tripling. But in the first trimester (up to 13 weeks), your need will probably *drop,* and you will have to keep adjusting your dose downward (with the help of your doctor) while watching out for hypoglycemic reactions. Reactions during these early weeks are very common and may occur without any warning, though medical consensus is that they won't hurt the baby. Don't make a move without your emergency sugar, be sure other people know how to handle possible reactions by giving you sugar or glucagon injections if you can't take it by mouth, and make certain your doctor is always available for consultation.

The dip in insulin need is probably due to the large amount of glucose the developing fetus and placenta are using, along with the effect of other hormonal changes, and perhaps morning sickness. You may not be eating (or keeping down) as much food as you usually do. Try to eat foods that appeal to you, space them out in small amounts throughout the day. This phase will soon pass and many women don't experience it at all. If necessary, your doctor may prescribe an antinausea drug. Or, when you can't keep anything down, drink three ounces of *regular* ginger ale every three hours until the nausea passes. Do not drink diet ginger ale. You will need the sugar in the soda. Besides, it is probably best to avoid unnecessary chemicals during pregnancy.

After the first two or three months, there is another big change. Now your insulin requirements start rising sharply and you must keep increasing your dose. Along with insulin shock, which remains a distinct possibility, you must be on the alert for the other extreme—acidosis. This, too, can come on very quickly now, and is a much more serious situation. If your tests are poor, if you have an infection, or if you are nauseated, very thirsty, breathless, or have any of the other symptoms of high sugar, check with your doctor immediately. Untreated, acidosis can be harmful to your baby.

Toward the end, around your eighth month, your insulin needs will probably stop rising and will level off.

After the baby is born, they will make another dramatic drop. You may not require any insulin for a few days, or much less than your usual dose. Then gradually, well within six weeks, you will return to your prepregnancy dose.

## SPLIT DOSES ARE BEST

Pregnant diabetics who require insulin do best with split doses, usually taking both quick-acting and Intermediate-acting insulin before breakfast and again before dinner. The Regular insulin takes care of breakfast and dinner; the Intermediate insulin takes care of lunch and the night, so that all bases are covered. In addition, you may need more shots if your sugar is high at any time during the day. You must respond to the information you get from your four daily blood-sugar tests.

If you never took insulin before your pregnancy, you probably won't need it after it's over. You may now return to your simple diet control or diet combined with oral agents. To return to oral agents, your doctor will probably ask you to take your prepregnancy dose and, if you have high sugar, to cover it with insulin before dinner and at bedtime. In a few days, you will know what your correct oral agent dose should be. If you are breast-feeding, do not go back to the pills until the baby is weaned.

## WHAT IS GOOD CONTROL?

Though other numbers may be tolerated when you are not pregnant, good control at this time translates to a blood-sugar level of *no lower than* 70 mgs, and *no higher than* 100 mgs fasting and 120 mgs two hours after a meal. This takes careful attention to your diet, and constant adjustments of your insulin if you require it. It also requires blood tests four times a day. It's surprising how many women, after playing fast and loose with their diabetes for years, become model patients when they are carrying a baby. Their concern for the baby makes them change their lifestyles radically, we hope forever.

You must check your blood four times a day, before breakfast, lunch, and bed, being sure to be accurate. Just to be safe, however, test for acetone when your sugar reads high. Acidosis is always a distinct possibility during pregnancy, and it may happen very quickly, so you must be constantly on the alert.

## USING THE INSULIN PUMP

In the few instances when a pregnant woman's diabetes continues to soar out of control despite her best efforts, doctors sometimes recommend an insulin pump (see page 122). This is a gadget worn around the waist. It infuses a few units of insulin per hour through a subcutaneous catheter and gives more before each meal, simulating the normal pancreatic output. Again, the goal is to maintain fasting sugar below 100 mgs and two hours after a meal no more than 120 mgs percent. Carefully attended, the pump can obviously provide excellent diabetic control.

## EATING FOR TWO

We haven't talked about total calories before, but now that you are pregnant, this becomes necessary. Most pregnant women require from 1,800 to 2,000 calories of food a day, but the amount that is right for you must be decided together with your doctor or a dietitian. Be sure to eat everything on your meal plan and eat it *on time*. When you strive to maintain the excellent blood-sugar control that is so important now, insulin reactions (if you are insulin-dependent) are always a possibility, even after the first trimester.

When you are pregnant, you will need more protein than at other times. Include two to five glasses of milk (skim or regular) during the day. You may also increase your usual meat portion at dinner.

Space your food throughout the day so your blood sugar doesn't rise and fall sharply. Your developing baby needs a constant supply of nutrients.

Take a daily multivitamin tablet that includes folic acid.

## "WILL MY BABY BE HEALTHY?"

If you're in good control and the baby is mature, your child has just about as good a chance of entering the world in as good condition as any other infant. The baby will not be born diabetic. In fact, there is a likelihood of hypoglycemia—low blood sugar—for a few hours or days after birth. While still in the uterus, the fetus was exposed to your blood sugar and the tiny pancreas responded by producing large amounts of insulin. A short period of time is needed now to settle down to normal. The pediatrician will have blood tests made to see if the baby requires supplements of sugar given by bottle or intravenously to compensate for the excessive insulin still being turned out.

Other possible results of the baby's long exposure to high sugar include low blood calcium and high blood bilirubin (which causes jaundice), neither of which is reason for serious concern today. Your pediatrician will be alerted to these complications and can correct them. Jaundice rarely needs more than a few days' exposure to ultraviolet lights, and low calcium is treated with intravenous calcium infusions. Babies born to diabetic mothers are usually kept in the nursery's intensive-care unit for a few days for close observation and, if necessary, treatment. Premature babies, of course, may require much longer hospital stays and special care by a team of neonatal specialists, but most infants are ready to go home with their mothers.

## "WILL MY BABY BE DIABETIC?"

Your baby will not be born diabetic. But, with a diabetic parent, there is a 1 percent chance your child will develop diabetes before the age of twenty and a 12 percent chance of developing it in its lifetime. Those are not overwhelming odds when you consider that 6 percent of the general population has the very same risk. With two diabetic parents, however, the chances rise to about 50 percent sometime in a life span.

By the way, a father who gets type 1 diabetes before the age of fifteen has a much greater chance of passing this disease along to a child than does a mother with type 1. But type 2 is different. Here the mother is the one who is more likely to have a child who develops type 2 diabetes.

## "DO DIABETIC COMPLICATIONS GET WORSE DURING A PREGNANCY?"

They could, especially if you do not maintain excellent control. On the other hand, they may improve. One study of a group of pregnant women with retinopathy reported that a third of the women were found to have improved by the time of delivery, a third stayed the same, and a third got worse. If your eyes happen to get worse, they can be treated with laser therapy at the onset to forestall further problems (see Chapter 11). It has been found, moreover, that eyes that become worse during pregnancy usually go back to their former condition afterwards.

Although kidney problems may increase during a pregnancy, women with mild kidney disease usually return to their prepregnant situation after their babies are born. However, for women with moderate-to-severe kidney disease, there is a 45 percent chance that pregnancy will make it worse, according to a recent study. In the meantime, kidney problems can make the pregnancy harder to manage.

## TIMING YOUR BABY'S ARRIVAL

Once it was true that many babies of diabetic mothers died in the last few weeks of pregnancy, and so it became customary to deliver the babies long before their due date. This led to problems. Because diabetic women sometimes have irregular periods, it wasn't easy to pinpoint the correct delivery time, and the babies were frequently brought into the world, usually by cesarean, before they were ready and suffered from all the problems associated with prematurity.

Today, however, sophisticated tests are available in most medical centers for measuring both fetal health and maturity. Every diabetic woman must be closely monitored, especially as she nears her due date, but Class A and Class B diabetics who do not have complications can often go all the way to term and deliver their babies in the usual fashion. More severe diabetics are delivered earlier, usually by the 38th week, but in most of these cases only after it has been determined that their babies are mature enough for this world. In these cases, labor is induced or a cesarean section is performed.

Many obstetricians put their diabetic patients into the hospital for their last two or three weeks, so they can be closely watched. Often, this is the best place to be.

How does the doctor know how your unborn baby is getting along? One way is to make frequent checks of your estriol levels toward the end of the pregnancy. A hormone produced by the fetal adrenal glands is changed to estriol by the placenta and excreted via the urine. The level normally rises continually throughout pregnancy and is an indication that the baby is doing well. But if the estriol level does not rise, or if it drops, then the doctor may decide the uterus no longer provides the best home for the baby and that it would be better off delivered early.

Estriol tests ideally should be made twice a week from the 30th week on in more severe cases, from the 35th week on in uncomplicated cases; then every day after you are hospitalized, just to be certain the baby is still safe.

The oxytocin challenge test is another way to find out if your unborn baby is healthy. In this procedure, the technician will fasten two belts around your abdomen, one which records the baby's heartbeat, the other your uterine contractions. You are given a small dose of oxytocin, which makes the uterus contract slightly, while the fetal heartbeat is watched to see if it remains normal.

Nonstress testing—monitoring the baby's heart rate—should start at the 30th or 32nd week of the pregnancy and will also help the doctor decide when the baby should be delivered.

## TESTING FOR MATURITY

Not many babies of diabetic mothers are delivered too early today, because now there are standard tests available at all large hospitals or in laboratories to determine whether they are mature enough to be born. The major problem of premature babies is respiratory distress syndrome (RDS), which means that the tiny lungs are not yet prepared to breathe air efficiently.

To predict lung maturity, amniotic fluid is tested for the presence of a substance called surfactant, which lines the air spaces of the lungs and helps in breathing. If enough surfactant is being produced, the baby's lungs are considered to be developed enough for delivery.

Sonography is another way to test for maturity. Pictures produced by sound waves, started very early in pregnancy, can monitor the rate of the baby's growth so that maturity can be estimated.

Sometimes the obstetrician will decide it is best to deliver your baby even though the lungs are not fully mature. In this case you may be given corticosteroids, which usually stimulate the production of enough surfactant within only 24 hours to ensure a safe delivery.

## "CAN I BREAST-FEED MY BABY?"

Being a diabetic mother doesn't affect your ability to breast-feed except that getting started may be a little more difficult if you are separated from your baby for very long after the birth. But even if you can't start immediately, it is quite possible to express your milk manually or with a pump so you will continue to produce it until you need it.

The baby will not be affected by the insulin you take, and won't have insulin reactions. You will probably require less insulin while you are breast-feeding because the baby is consuming some of your glucose supply in the milk, so be alert to your own possible reactions and make adjustments in your dosage if your sugar tends to fall very low.

Because breast-feeding can cause rapid drops in glucose levels, be sure to have a carbohydrate snack before each nursing session.

You must also adjust your diet, adding about 600 to 900 calories a day to compensate for the amount you are expending. Extra milk is an excellent way to get those calories.

Remember that you must not take oral agents while you are breast-feeding. If diet isn't doing the job of controlling your blood sugar, you must take insulin temporarily.

## COW'S MILK OR BREAST MILK?

It was once thought that babies who drink cow's milk have an increased risk of developing diabetes. But not to worry. Recent research at the University of Colorado School of Medicine in Denver found that early exposure to cow's milk is not associated with beta-cell autoimmunity, an early predictor of type 1 diabetes.

# 15

# SEX AND THE DIABETIC

Does being diabetic affect your sex life? It can, especially if you are a man. It is estimated that about a quarter of middle-aged diabetic men who have had the disease for many years, who suffer from neuropathy, and probably have not maintained very good control, become impotent. Though sexual difficulties can obviously be psychological (and often the anxiety about the possibility of future problems can cause them), in most cases an organic disfunction quite specific to diabetes is the reason for an increased incidence of impotence at an earlier age than the rest of the population.

What occurs is not loss of libido or desire for sexual gratification, but the ability to have an erection. This ability may gradually diminish and eventually vanish completely. Usually the cause is neuropathy damage to the nerves responsible for stimulating the arteries in the penis to dilate and produce an erection. This is almost always associated with other neuropathies, often in the legs and feet and, most likely, the bladder.

Occasionally the reason is an obstruction or clot in one of the blood vessels supplying the penis, and sometimes poorly controlled diabetes causes temporary impotence as a result of a general weakened condition.

## POSSIBILITY OF IMPOTENCE

Though some studies have been made, it is still uncertain just how many diabetic men eventually develop sexual problems by middle age. Uncertain, too, is whether impotence is related to the severity of the diabetes. Undoubtedly it is affected by the quality of blood-sugar control over the years, and the number of years since the diagnosis was made.

This does not mean that impotence is in the cards for every male diabetic—there are men who have had diabetes for fifty years and have no problem—nor that all is lost and nothing can be done about it.

First, it must be determined whether your impotence, which never happens suddenly but comes about gradually when it is caused by diabetes, is psychological or physiological. Your internist will suggest an examination by a urologist and perhaps a neurologist, and if there is no obvious physical reason for the problem, may suggest an NPT (nocturnal penile tumescence) assessment. This is usually performed in the sleep-disorder department of a large medical center, and monitors the nocturnal erections that normally occur at regular intervals while a man sleeps. If you have normal nocturnal erections, then you are not suffering from nerve or vascular damage and psychological counseling will probably be recommended. If your neuropathy is the culprit, you will not have erections in your sleep or at any other time.

Obviously, if your impotence is the result of poor diabetic control, then good control is your answer.

If the cause is vascular obstruction, sometimes surgery can make a dramatic difference.

## DEALING WITH IMPOTENCE

When impotence is caused by neuropathy, there is a choice of treatments available today and one of them may work for you. First, ask your doctor to check your testosterone level to see if you are producing a normal amount. If not, you can take supplemental testosterone by mouth, injection, or skin patch (Androderm) and see if it enhances your libido and the ability to maintain an erection.

Other remedies include drugs, implants, injections, pumps, and more. A urologist who specializes in problems of impotency can explain the merits of each and the possibilities that one of them will be helpful for you. One recently F.D.A.-approved treatment is Muse (alprostadil or prostaglandin E-1), a drug that is delivered by means of a plastic applicator that inserts a pellet into the urethral opening of the penis. In laboratory tests, two thirds of the men who tried it achieved sexual intercourse. This drug may also be injected into the base of the penis just before intercourse.

Viagra is the trade name for another drug called sildenafil that is taken by pill about an hour before it is needed and enhances the response to sexual stimulation. In a study of more than 350 users, 65 to 88 percent reported improved erections. If proven to be free of side effects, this drug will surely be a boon to many men.

And finally, yohimbine, available as an herb or a prescription drug, has been found to be useful in some cases.

Though there is no way to repair damaged nerve endings, you may want to look into the possibility of a penile implant or an inflatable device, both of which are designed to allow sexual intercourse complete with ejaculation and orgasm. When you have an implant, flexible silicone rods are placed in the penis, making it rigid enough for intercourse. A problem is that the penis remains rigid.

The more complex "inflatable erectile prosthesis" allows actual simulation of a natural erection by the implantation of a device that inflates and deflates the penis on demand by squeezing a pump.

Another possible helpful aid is a vacuum constriction device that gives the penis rigidity. This is a noninvasive technique and may be worth a try before resorting to implants.

## EFFECTS ON FERTILITY

Diabetes doesn't affect a man's ability to produce sperm, so, assuming he is not impotent, there's usually no reason he cannot father children. Sometimes, though, diabetic neuropathy will cause a condition known as "retrograde ejaculation." Because the nerve supply to the penis is impaired, the sphincters won't open and the semen, including the sperm, drops back into the bladder. This doesn't interfere with intercourse or orgasm, but obviously precludes fertility.

## SEX AND THE DIABETIC WOMAN

Diabetic women tend to have more sexual difficulties than women with normal blood sugar, often experiencing a marked reduction in lubrication and sometimes in their sexual desire and ability to have orgasms. This is especially true when they have peripheral nerve damage which diminishes sensation. If you are experiencing such problems, try taking vitamin B complex every day and asking your doctor about the new drugs now available for treating neuropathy (see Chapter 11).

Women with diabetes may also have other related problems as a result of lowered glucose tolerance.

One is an increased tendency toward vaginal and urinary infections. The high sugar environment when you are in less-than-ideal control promotes the growth of bacteria and yeast. Yeast especially loves the glucose found in vaginal secretions and many a case of diabetes has been first detected in the gynecologist's office. Add to that the sometimes diminished ability of the white cells to rally around and fight infections. If you notice any signs of vaginal or urinary infection, get yourself to your doctor immediately. There are drugs that can alleviate them, usually in short order. Along with the drugs, however, you must get your diabetes back in good control and keep it there.

Vaginal dryness is another problem that often accompanies poorly controlled diabetes. This will improve along with better control and, in the meantime, can be counteracted by the use of a personal lubricant made for this purpose, such as K-Y Jelly, Astroglide, or Surgilube. By the way, never use a lubricant that is not designed for vaginal use. Most cosmetic creams, for example, contain ingredients that can irritate tender tissues. Don't use petroleum jelly or oil because it may cake and dry, provide a habitat for bacteria, and block the release of your own secretions as well. The only exception is vitamin E oil, which doesn't dry and may possibly have a beneficial effect on the vaginal lining.

Even more effective than lubricants are nonhormonal vaginal moisturizing gels, including Replens and Gyne-Moistrin, now sold over the counter. They help by plumping up the cells of the lining with moisture, making it less dry and irritable. They should not be used as lubricants, however, but inserted into the vagina about three times a week, preferably in the morning. If you need a lubricant, too, use it just before intercourse.

## WHAT KIND OF CONTRACEPTION?

For the diabetic, probably the best countraceptive methods are the mechanical kinds—the diaphragm or the condom. These usually present no problems, as long as you remember to use them every time, unless you are prone to fungal infections. If you do get these infections frequently, try using a condom with a spermicidal foam that has an acidic component to discourage fungus.

Birth-control pills are not the best idea for several reasons. Most important, some studies have shown that the hormones in the pill can lower your glucose tolerance and raise your insulin needs. If you do use them, choose combination estrogen-progesterone pills with the lowest dose and potency of progestin available. Keep a close watch on your glucose to be sure it is not affected and stay in touch with your doctors.

Many physicians think that the IUD, the intrauterine device, is associated with increased vaginal infections. Diabetics need no more ways of acquiring infections. In addition, according to researchers, there is a high failure (pregnancy) rate among diabetic IUD users, probably because of an unusual metabolic interaction of the device with the endometrium, the uterine lining.

For those couples who do not want children or have completed their families, sterilization is an option.

## CHANGES IN INSULIN NEEDS

For many women, insulin requirements change the week before their menstrual period, so you should check your blood and respond accordingly. Your pattern of needing more or less insulin at that time will usually remain consistent.

## IF YOU USE AN INSULIN PUMP

Obviously, it may be uncomfortable to have sexual intercourse while wearing an insulin pump. If you can't find a satisfactory position, it won't hurt you to detach it for a while, just as you do when you take a bath.

## HORMONE REPLACEMENT AFTER MENOPAUSE

A few years back, hormone replacement therapy (HRT) after menopause was considered out of the question for diabetic women. Not true anymore. Because the estrogen dose in HRT is so tiny today, it rarely affects sugar metabolism, according to Lila Nachtigall, M.D., of New York University Medical Center, author of *Estrogen: The Facts Can Change Your Life* (HarperCollins, 1995). Unless there are real contraindications, such as an abnormal clotting condition, you should seriously consider taking estrogen because it will help keep your heart and arteries healthier, your bones sturdier, and your vagina in good condition. Coronary heart disease is the diabetic's major health risk.

Another reason to consider HRT is early menopause. Type 1 diabetics often have premature menopause, sometimes even before the age of forty, giving them more time to develop health problems associated with estrogen deficiency.

Take your estrogen by transdermal patch, rather than by mouth. Taking it orally can increase your risk of gallbladder disease, a problem diabetics already face without any help from the outside. When you absorb the hormone through the skin instead of the digestive system, that increased risk is avoided. And watch for new developments in the kinds of estrogen available. Currently under investigation are "designer estrogens" with new characteristics.

# 16

# TRAVELING: DIABETICS ON THE MOVE

If you are just a beginner at this business of being a diabetic, you probably are afraid to travel. You feel much safer at home. You are not interested in surprises, not when you're away from your own kitchen, your own medicine cabinet, and especially your own doctor.

But once you have learned the rules, whether it involves only diet or includes insulin or pills, and you have had sufficient practice coping with the variations of a diabetic life, then there is no reason you cannot travel anywhere in this world like anyone else. But you must remember, just because you're breathing the pure mountain air of the Alps or savoring the sights of Hong Kong, you have not left your diabetes behind you. It travels with you. So the same rules apply wherever you are.

There are a few precautions that a person with diabetes, especially one who is insulin-dependent, should take. Let's run through them briefly. If you are not yet an experienced traveler, you may want to slip this book into your luggage for handy reference.

## A BEFORE-YOU-GO LIST OF SUGGESTIONS

• Don't travel (and that means anywhere, including the next town) without some visible medical identification affixed to your person. Wear a bracelet or necklace stating "I am a diabetic," and carry two cards (one in your pocket, another in your wallet) that say the same and also list your medication and allergies, along with your name, address, and phone number. If possible, carry a card in the language of the country you are visiting.

• Before leaving town, go to your doctor for a checkup to be sure you are in good shape for your venture. Don't go anywhere when your condition isn't stable. Get checked out by your dentist too, so that you don't find yourself in Afghanistan with a toothache and a blood-sugar level that's askew. Go to your podiatrist, because you will undoubtedly be doing a lot of walking and you should be sure there is no foot trouble brewing.

• Take along an extra pair of eyeglasses, or a least a copy of your prescription. Many a person, not necessarily diabetic, has toured Europe out of focus after losing his/her only pair of glasses the first week out.

• Have any necessary innoculations long before your departure date, so any reactions to them will be over before your trip. Sometimes the shots affect your diabetic equilibrium.

## BE PREPARED FOR PROBLEMS

• Ask your doctor to prescribe an antidiarrheal medication to take along, just in case you'll need it. Lomotil and Immodium are effective for treating the symptoms. Antibiotics such as Bactrim or Cipro will help prevent or treat the disease itself.

If you are going to a country where you are fairly sure to run into intestinal problems, pack some Pepto-Bismol tablets and take one tablet four times a day as a preventive. Don't be frightened if your tongue and stool turn black.

Also take along an antiemetic to prevent or treat nausea. If you are susceptible to motion sickness, take the preventive four hours *before* you board the boat, walk into the airplane, or step into the car. Be sure to take along some antiemetic medication in suppository form in case you can't keep anything down. Remember, too, that medicine like Compazine, effective against nausea, can be injected with your insulin syringe.

• Carry in your pocket or handbag a signed note from your physician stating that you are a diabetic and require insulin and syringes. That's so the customs inspectors, coming upon a supply of syringes, won't suspect they have discovered a drug addict who must be turned over to the *gendarmes*. The statement will also help you buy more syringes if you need them. Make sure the note explains your current treatment and lists any other medications you take in addition to insulin.

• Take more than enough oral agents or insulin and syringes *for the entire trip*. Always include a bottle of Regular fast-acting insulin, even if you normally take only Intermediate insulin or none at all. In an emergency, this will be essential.

• A pen injector or a syringe prefilled with insulin may be more convenient when you're on the move.

• Take plenty of blood-glucose testing equipment. Although you may prefer the strip tests for traveling, it's best to take a glucose meter and use it to test your blood as usual. Meters are small and light today.

• If you use an insulin pump, include extra pump supplies and don't forget the user manual. Talk to your doctor about resetting the pump if you are changing time zones. Just in case, take insulin and syringes too.

• Try a hospital emergency room if you have problems getting supplies away from home.

## DON'T BE CAUGHT SHORT

• Unopened insulin need not be refrigerated. It will survive nicely for a few months in any environment that's comfortable for you. Do not use insulin that has been exposed to very hot temperatures (don't let it sit in the sun or in a closed car) or has been frozen. This means it must *not* be packed in your luggage if you fly, because temperatures are often below freezing in the baggage compartments. Oral hypoglycemic agents are not harmed by freezing, however.

• Carry your oral agents or insulin and syringes *with you* in your hand luggage to cover those possible occasions when you go one way and your luggage goes another. This is important. It won't be harmed by the airport X-ray machines. Disposable insulin syringes may be used more than once. Seven syringes can be adequate for two weeks. After use, simply recap the needle. Also carry *with you* your insulin pump infusion sets, lancets, glucose meter, glucagon kit, glucose gel or tablets, blood and ketone test strips. And don't forget some snacks.

• If you take insulin, carrying your own is especially important. In many countries, only U-40 is available. But don't panic if you run short—it's really quite simple to convert your usual dose to U-40 (see Chapter 7).

• Your brand of insulin will probably be available in other countries, but it may help to know that, in Europe, Regular or fast-acting insulin is often called Actrapid. Rapitard or Lentard or Monotard would correspond to our NPH or Lente insulins. Ultratard would be equivalent to Ultralente. In most cases, the dose would be the same or slightly less than your accustomed dose of nonmonocomponent insulin.

You may want to write or call the manufacturer of the insulin you use (well before your departure date) to ask about its availability and its trade names in the countries you will be visiting. You can avoid all problems by carrying more than enough of your own with you.

• A good thing to remember is that 1-cc tuberculin syringes can be substituted for U-100 syringes where each line equals one unit of insulin.

• If you take oral agents and need to buy more, you will find counterparts available in foreign countries.

## SPEAKING THEIR LANGUAGE

• If you are going somewhere where a language other than your own is spoken, memorize in the appropriate language (and write in clear lettering on a card) the following phrases: "I am a diabetic." "Sugar or orange juice, please." "Please get me a doctor."

Here they are in four languages:

*I am a diabetic.*
French: *Je suis diabétique.*
Spanish: *Yo soy diabético.*
German: *Ich bin zuckerkrank.*
Italian: *Io sono diabètico.*

*Sugar or orange juice, please.*
French: *Sucre ou jus d'orange, s'il vous plaît.*
Spanish: *Azúcar o un vaso de jugo de naranja, por favor.*
German: *Zucker oder Orangensaft, bitte.*
Italian: *Zucchero o succo di arància, per favore.*

*Please get me a doctor.*
French: *Allez chercher un médecin, si'il vous plaît.*
Spanish: *Haga me el favor de llamar al médico.*
German: *Rufen Sie bitte einen Arzt.*
Italian: *Per favore chiami un dottore.*

• Another precaution before you leave home: Though you certainly hope it won't happen in the middle of a great vacation, there's always the possibility of getting sick and needing a doctor, whether you are diabetic or not. It is always best to be prepared. Write to the American Diabetes Association (1660 Duke Street, Alexandria, VA 22314) or call 800-342-2383 for a list of affiliate or chapter offices of the Association wherever you plan to travel within the United States. If you need a doctor in Cleveland, for example, a call to the Cleveland Diabetes Association will get you a list of local doctors experienced in diabetic care.

From the same national ADA office or from the British Diabetic Association (10 Queen Anne Street, London W1M OBD, England) you can get a list of diabetes associations in foreign countries. (Telephone: London 011-44-171-637-3644.)

When you arrive at your destination, remember that the U.S. embassy or consulate will supply the names of English-speaking physicians upon request. So will the major hotels.

Another suggestion: Well before you leave on a trip to a foreign country, send for a list of English-speaking physicians all over the world, and information on climate, food, and sanitary conditions from the free, nonprofit International Association for Medical Assistance to Travellers (IAMAT, 417 Center Street, Lewiston, NY 14092. Telephone: 716-754-4883).

## TRAVEL TIPS ON YOUR WAY

Now you have finally had all the proper checkups, your diabetes is under excellent control, you have gathered your supplies together, tucked away all those lists and statements. You are ready to get your show on the road. *And* you do not want to hear any more advice. However, we have a few more tips, all designed to make it easier for the traveler who happens to have diabetes.

## CHANGING TIME ZONES

Most people who take medication for diabetes are concerned about their schedules for insulin or pills when they cross time zones (traveling north or south requires no adjustments). When you travel by car or ship, no problem. The time changes are so gradual they will not affect your timetable. Simply take your medication at your usual hour according to the time it is wherever you are.

If you take oral agents, do the same, even if you fly long distances, crossing many time zones. Take the pills according to your new time.

But when you fly long distances into new time zones and you take insulin, it gets a little trickier. Here's how to handle it.

Keep your watch set at your point-of-departure time, so you will know how many hours have passed since your last injection. Eat your meals and snacks on your normal schedule, according to the time on your watch. If you have requested special meals or mealtimes when you made your reservations, confirm this 24 hours before the flight, and remind the flight attendant when you board the plane that you must have your meals on time because you are a diabetic. If meals at different times from those of the other passengers seem to be too difficult to arrange, board the plane with your own box of food. (And, of course, you have not set forth without your usual emergency snack supplies.)

On arrival, if *more* than 24 hours have passed since your last injection, take a few *extra* units of Regular insulin and/or Intermediate insulin. However, if *less* than 24 hours have passed since your last injection, take *fewer* units of Intermediate-acting insulin because some of the dose you took the previous day is still in your bloodstream. If you are skipping a meal, you must adjust for less food.

After taking your insulin, set your watch to the time of the place in which you now find yourself, and start taking your injections accordingly.

## GOING FROM WEST TO EAST

When you are traveling east, perhaps from the United States to Europe, your day will be *less* than 24 hours long and you will require less insulin. Suppose you have your insulin shot at 7 A.M. on the day of departure. You leave New York at 6 P.M. and arrive in Europe at 2 A.M. our time. But it is 8 A.M. European time. Breakfast will have been served on the plane before landing. Do not eat it. And do not take your morning insulin at that time. Instead, take it at noon just before lunch when it is about 24 hours from the time you took your last shot.

Do not take your second shot before dinner because your day has been condensed and you don't want to overdose—you could end up in the hospital with an insulin reaction instead of on a tour bus having a fine time.

Now set your watch to European time. The next morning, take your usual dose.

Remember to adjust your insulin to your physical activity. If you will be much more active than you normally are at home, you must compensate by taking a few less units of insulin or eating more food (see Chapter 5).

## GOING FROM EAST TO WEST

Now, what about going the other way, from east to west when your first day of travel will be *more* than 24 hours? Let's use this example: You take your insulin and depart from Europe at 8 A.M. You arrive in New York seven hours later at 3 P.M. European time, 10 A.M. New York time.

Keep your watch set on foreign time. You have had breakfast before getting on the plane, and you have eaten lunch during the flight. Your next meal is dinner at 6 P.M. European time but noon in New York. Eat your dinner then. Eat your bedtime snack at 11 P.M. European time, 7 P.M. in New York.

Go to bed early. When you wake up, you are five hours late for your next shot. Take a little more of your Regular insulin and the usual dose of NPH or Lente. If you are not on Regular insulin, take your usual dose of NPH or Lente and eat less starch for breakfast.

• Never make a move without your cache of emergency carbohydrates. You must have this *with* you at all times, just on the chance—however remote it may be in your case—that you will have a hypoglycemic reaction. Sugar cubes, candies, cookies, crackers. Don't carry sugar-free candies; they won't help you a bit if you have low blood sugar.

• If you are traveling by car, and especially if you are the driver, take the equivalent of 10 grams of carbohydrate every hour: two graham crackers, an orange, 15 grapes, whatever.

## NOW YOU ARE THERE

Once you have arrived at your destination, simply start living in your accustomed way, adjusting your medication to your blood-sugar level and your physical activity just as you would at home.

A few things to keep in mind:

• You may be much more active on vacation than you are in everyday life. If you are going to do strenuous sightseeing, play tennis, ski, swim, anything that burns up considerable sugar, you will require more food or less insulin. Oral agents are not so critical and do not have to be adjusted. On the other hand, if you overindulge, you cannot expect an extra pill to correct it, as you would if you were on insulin and took an extra dose when your sugar was high.

Suppose you plan to play a few tough sets of singles, make a cross-country ski trek, or even do some heavy sightseeing on foot.

Check your blood. If it is low, eat extra carbohydrate and protein before setting off. If it is high, have some carbohydrate after about an hour of exercise. Or reduce your insulin as an added precaution against reactions. Sometimes you will need snacks every half hour or so of heavy exercise. Try to avoid strenuous exercise when your insulin is peaking (see Chapter 5).

• Never ski, swim, bike, hike, or climb alone, but always rely on the buddy system. If you should have a reaction, your buddy will cope with it. Unless you started off with high sugar, the exertion may drop your blood sugar very quickly to subnormal levels.

• At high altitudes, the symptoms of altitude mountain sickness (AMS) can mimic those of hypoglycemic reactions, perhaps making you feel lightheaded, weak, confused, shaky, breathless. Are you suffering from AMS or low sugar? You will know only by testing your sugar at that very moment.

· Be prepared for delays when you travel. You never know when a traffic jam, a delayed flight, or a missed connection will mess up your schedule. Carry some snacks and drinks with you. Be prepared to make adjustments in your medication and meals.

## KEEP YOUR SHOES ON!

· Remember if you have foot problems not to go barefoot, even on the beach. One sharp shell can get you into long-term trouble. Don't get sunburned. A burn is a burn, and the stress it causes can throw off your control.

Use foot powder, wash your feet, and change your socks frequently. Keep an eye on your feet, giving them a daily inspection. Unaccustomed walking can produce blisters and rubs, especially if you are wearing new shoes, which you should *not* be doing. Do not let any foot injuries get even the slightest bit out of control. Rest your feet, take the pressure off, wear sneakers, sandals, or slippers if necessary, and if trouble seems to be brewing, see a doctor *immediately*, not two weeks after you have returned home.

· Watch what you eat. Nobody wants a gastrointestinal upset, but diabetics can have their whole vacation ruined by the after-effects and the difficulty of getting their blood sugar back under control. In tropical countries, don't eat raw vegetables, soft cheese, ice cream, rare meats, cream sauces, fruits you can't peel. Use bottled or boiled water even for brushing your teeth. Don't drink fresh milk or water, and avoid ice cubes. One man bought an unpeeled melon in India, thinking he could eat it safely once it was skinned. But his host served it to him cut up and floating in ice water. He had his melon, plus a good case of amebiasis and diarrhea.

· If you get up late and miss breakfast, take about 20 percent less insulin because you'll be having only two meals that day. Don't try to make up for the lost meal by eating more now, because that will present you with too much carbohydrate to handle at one time.

## DINING FASHIONABLY LATE

• In some countries—Spain, for example—the dinner hour is late. If you plan to have your meal at the fashionable hour of, say, 10 P.M., then you must prepare in advance. There are two ways to handle this situation. Either take less insulin in the morning and give yourself a second shot before going to bed. Or consume the major portion of your carbohydrate allowance (the equivalent of two slices of bread) at 6 P.M., then eat everything else—your main course, vegetables, dessert— at dinner. Of course, you will then skip the carbohydrates at the table—rice, corn, potatoes, bread, etc. And don't eat your bedtime snack either. This also applies to weddings and other parties here at home.

• Be sure your traveling companions know how to cope with both hypoglycemia (low sugar) and hyperglycemia (high sugar). Your companions should know that you need quick sugar if you are having an insulin reaction—granulated sugar, honey, a soft drink (not a diet drink), candy, orange juice, etc., followed shortly thereafter by some protein. Or you may be given "instant glucose" or cake icing, which comes in toothpastelike tubes and can be forced through the lips. If this isn't quickly effective, a subcutaneous shot of glucagon and a doctor may be necessary. Have all the supplies always handy (see Chapter 9).

If you are suffering from *high* sugar *and* acetone, then you need insulin and perhaps the service of a doctor.

• Adjust the eating customs of the places you visit to your own needs. This means making sure you get the right proportions of carbohydrate, protein, and fat, no matter where you are. A continental breakfast, for example—a roll and coffee—isn't going to be enough for you unless that is what you normally consume at home. Order additional food. Many foods, notably a lot of Chinese and Japanese dishes, contain sugar and must be avoided. Sukiyaki, for example, is made with sugar or sweet wine.

Remember your carbohydrate exchanges: 1 cup of rice is the equivalent of 2 slices of bread, or 30 grams of carbohydrate. So is one regular-size pita, even if it is flat as a pancake. Some tropical fruits, such as mangos, are very high in sugar. Check them out before eating them freely.

• Test your blood glucose after you've eaten a food that you're not accustomed to eating. If the effect is to raise your sugar inordinately, avoid that food in the future.

• Wines and liquors needn't be avoided, if you drink them in moderation, as you do at home (see pages 75–78).

• If you happen to get sick away from home, treat yourself just as you would in your natural habitat (see Chapter 12). Test your blood four times a day for sugar and if it's high, check your urine for acetone. *Always take your insulin.* If your sugar is low *and* you can't eat, take half your usual dose of insulin. If your sugar is high, whether you can eat or not, take your regular amount. Always take your normal dosage of oral agents unless your sugar is very low, under 100 mgs.

If you have high sugar and are vomiting, take your full insulin dose. Then take an antiemetic by suppository. Eat or drink some carbohydrate every hour—perhaps 3 ounces of orange juice mixed with water, or 3 ounces of ginger ale (*not* sugar-free), or ice cream, toast, broth, cereal, etc. Don't tough it out—if you need a doctor, get one.


## TRAVELING IS FUN, REMEMBER?

With all these precautions and pieces of advice, perhaps you think it might be simpler to stay home. But make all your preparations, keep the advice in the back of your mind just in case you need it, and go forth, not to worry, but to enjoy yourself. You take your diabetes with you, but other people take their problems with them, too, and may not be as carefree as they seem. Enjoy.

# 17

# CAN DIABETES
# BE PREVENTED?

Is it possible that diabetes can be prevented or at least delayed by medications, diet and exercise, vitamins, or insulin
pills? Current thinking is that the risk of developing either
type 1 or type 2 diabetes can definitely be decreased and
teams of researchers are now testing ways to do it. Too late
for you, but your family members may be able to avoid this
disease if they heed the results.

For example, researchers conducting a nationwide study
sponsored by the National Institutes of Health are now trying
to determine whether taking capsules of insulin crystals by
mouth or small daily doses of injected insulin can prevent or
postpone the disease for those most at risk for type 1 diabetes—children and young adults with a diabetic parent or
sibling.

Volunteers for the study are between three and forty-five
years old and immediate relatives of a person with type 1, or
more distant relatives between the ages of three and twenty.
The volunteers have been randomly assigned to three groups,
with one taking insulin shots, another swallowing daily capsules of insulin crystals, and the third acting as a control
group taking placebos.

The theory is that by giving insulin by capsules or injections to susceptible people before they develop the disease, it may be possible to stop the body's immune system from attacking the pancreas and destroying its beta cells. The results of the study have the potential to change many lives.

## WHO WILL GET TYPE 1?

Those at special risk for developing type 1 (IDDM or juvenile-onset) can be identified by their genetic characteristics. Children with the genes DR3 or DR4 on their sixth chromosomes, for example, have 2½ times more chance of becoming diabetic after a viral infection. Eighty-five to 90 percent of all type 1 diabetics have DR3 and/or DR4.

Another indicator of high risk is the presence of one or more kinds of antibodies in the bloodstream: islet-cell antibodies, ILA2 antibodies, or GAD 65 antibodies. With all three of these antibodies, the likelihood of developing diabetes within two years is almost 100 percent; with two of the antibodies, it's 80 percent.

## PREVENTING TYPE 2

Twenty-five medical centers across the country are participating in a six-year Diabetes Prevention Program focused on preventing or delaying the onset of type 2 (NIDDM or adult-onset) diabetes in volunteers who have been deemed at high risk. This means they have impaired glucose tolerance and higher than normal blood-sugar levels but not high enough to be classified as diabetes. Risk factors for IGT include obesity, a family history of diabetes, or a history of gestational diabetes while pregnant. It is already known that about half of the people with impaired glucose tolerance will eventually develop diabetes and the hope is that early treatment can make a difference.

The volunteers, over 4,000 of them, are assigned to one of four treatments: one group emphasizes intensive lifestyle factors including thirty minutes of exercise daily; another is treated with the diabetes drug metformin (Glucophage); a third receives the drug troglitazone (Rezulin); and the fourth group gets a placebo.

In the meantime, the hunt for genes that cause type 2 diabetes continues. One group of scientists is participating in the Gennid Study at eight Harold Rifkin Family Acquisition Centers around the country in an effort to map the responsible genes. And researchers at the Johns Hopkins University School of Medicine are investigating the genetic link by studying a gene mutation that is thought to promote the development of both type 2 and obesity.

## CAN SUSCEPTIBLE PEOPLE AVOID DIABETES?

It is believed that type 2 is caused by a combination of genes and lifestyle, so it makes great sense for genetically susceptible individuals to make certain changes in their everyday lives. Here is our advice to your family members and friends who are at risk:

### Keep your weight down.

The most important change you can make is to lose weight if you are too heavy, especially if you carry much of the extra fat around your middle. A weight loss of 11 to 44 pounds can reduce the risk of diabetes by 30 percent in just four years, according to the findings of the ongoing Nurses' Health Study that is following the health of some 114,000 women.

### Exercise.

You can reduce your risk of developing adult diabetes by exercise, which improves the body's ability to metabolize sugar. In a study by epidemiologists at the University of California at Berkeley, middle-aged men were found to decrease their risk by 6 percent with every 500 calories they burned each week. Men who were very active, burning about 3,500 calories a week, cut their risk in half when compared with men who were sedentary.

*Improve your diet.*

The content of your diet is also a factor, with high fat intake predisposing to the development of impaired glucose tolerance, according to some experts. Replace the fat with more whole grains and fiber. A recent report from the Nurses' Health Study emphasizes the importance of dietary fiber in fending off type 2. It found that the women who ate more fiber, especially more fiber from cereal (and especially cold cereal) with minimally processed grains, had a lower risk of diabetes. The reason may be that less-refined foods are less rapidly digested and so enter the system more slowly, lowering insulin secretion and placing less stress on the pancreas.

*Be cautious with diuretics.*

Diuretics, usually taken for hypertension, have the potential of lowering insulin sensitivity, thereby increasing the risk of developing diabetes in some people. Because this tendency may be related to low potassium levels, it may make sense, if your doctor deems water pills a necessity, to take a potassium supplement. Even better would be to ask your doctor about other blood-pressure medications.

*Consider alcohol.*

The latest apparent benefit of alcohol is an improved insulin response. That can lead to decreased secretion of insulin and to lower blood-sugar levels. This may explain the fact that moderate drinkers are less likely to develop diabetes than nondrinkers, according to two large studies. Moderate drinking may also boost HDL, the "good" cholesterol, and help protect your heart.

# RESOURCES

For additional information and help, here is a list of resources that will answer questions, send general information and literature, and provide referrals as well as the addresses and telephone numbers of their local affiliates or chapters.

American Diabetes Association, 1660 Duke Street, Alexandria, VA 22314; 800-342-2383.

International Diabetes Federation, 40 Washington Street, B-1050, Brussels, Belgium.

Juvenile Diabetes Foundation, 120 Wall Street, New York, NY 10005; 800-223-1138.

National Diabetes Information Clearing House, National Institutes of Health, 1 Information Way, Bethesda, MD 20892; 301-654-3327.

Diabetes Control Network, 800-DCN-5554.

MedicAlert, 800-344-3226.

International Association for Medical Assistance to Travellers (IAMAT), 417 Center Street, Lewiston, NY 14092; 716-754-4883.

The Lighthouse, 111 East 59 Street, New York, NY 10022; 800-334-5497.

"The Diabetic Traveler," a quarterly newsletter that addresses the special concerns of diabetics away from home or on the road, PO Box 8223-Rw, Stamford, CT 06905; 203-327-5832.

# INDEX

acarbose, 96, 100, 101
ACE inhibitors, 175
acetone (ketones), 8, 237
  testing for, 135–36
  testing for while sick, 189
acidophilis tablets, 193
acidosis, 10, 79, 88, 153–57, 190,
    191
  causes of, 155–56
  defined, 154
  insulin reactions vs., 151–52
  during pregnancy, 212
  prevention of, 157
  symptoms of, 154
  treatment of, 156–57
Actos, 100, 101
Actrapid, 230
adrenal imbalance, 12
"adult-onset" diabetes. See type 2
    diabetes
African Americans
  incidence of diabetes in, 5, 158,
    165
  kidney problems in, 175
age of onset
  type 1, 10
  type 2, 9

Albert Einstein College of Medi-
    cine, 182
alcohol consumption, 73, 238
  effect on cholesterol levels, 163
  exercise and, 93–94
  guidelines to follow, 75–76, 78
  hypoglycemia due to, 20, 22
  insulin reactions and, 147
  moderate, benefits of, 242
alcoholic drinks, 73, 77
allergic reactions to insulin, 116
alpha cells, 7
alprostadil, 222
ALT 462/ALT 480, 160
altitude mountain sickness (AMS),
    235–36
Amaryl, 96, 98, 101
amebiasis, 236
American Diabetes Association
    (ADA), 15, 26, 29, 97, 138,
    189, 208, 231
American Medical Association
    (AMA), 97
Americans, rates of diabetes
    among, 5
aminoguanidine, 160, 175
amphetamines, 75

amputations, 13, 197
amylin, 7
amyloid, 160
Androderm, 222
1,5-anhydroglucitol, 141
Antabuse effect, 76, 78, 98
antibiotics, tendency to fungal
    infections and, 185, 193
antibodies, risk of developing type
    1 and, 240
antidepressants, 177
antidiabetic agents, 19
apples, 58
applesauce, 58
arteriosclerosis, 161–62
    prevention of, Amaryl and, 98
artificial sweeteners, 60, 71–72
Asians, rates of diabetes among, 5
aspartame (Nutrasweet, Equal,
    Sweetmate, NutraTaste), 72
aspirin, 164–65
atherosclerosis, cholesterol and, 56
athlete's foot, 185, 198
Atkins diet, 79
Avandia, 100, 101
avocados, 43

bacon, 47
bagels, 47
bananas, 46, 57
Banting, Frederick, 107–8
bathing, 187
beans, 68
bedtime insulin/daytime sulfonyl-
    ureas (BIDS), 106
beer, 76
Benemid, 195
Best, Charles, 107–8
beta blockers, 147
beta cells, 7, 10, 109
beta-cell autoimmunity, 219
BIDS, 106
biguanides, 99
birth-control pills, 224

bladder, effect of neuropathy on,
    179
bladder infections, 179–80, 223
blindness, 13
blisters, diabetic, 187
blood clots, dissolving, exercise
    and, 85
blood pressure. See hypertension
blood sugar levels in diabetics, 5,
    28, 29
    control of, in preventing compli-
        cations, 13–14, 159, 167, 182,
        213–14
    effect of exercise on, 84
    hormonal regulation of, 7
    influence of carbohydrates on,
        36–39, 40
    low. See hypoglycemia
    normal fasting, 7, 17–18, 28, 29,
        132
    sickness and, 134, 189
    testing of, 130–34, 136–41
    testing while traveling, 229
blood tests, 130–34, 136–41
    with blood-glucose meters,
        138–39
    fasting plasma glucose test, 26
    frequency of, 132–33
    fructosamine test, 140–41
    glucose tolerance test (GTT), 25,
        27
    glycosuria and renal thresholds,
        131–32
    HbA1c: the glycohemoglobin
        test, 26–27, 139–40
    home methods, 136–37
    importance of, 131
    record keeping for, 133–34
    sickness and, 134, 189
    with a strip, 137–38
    while traveling, 229
blood-glucose meters, 138–39
blurred vision, 147, 171–72
body mass index (BMI), 52

bran, 67–68
breaded foods, 61
breads, 46, 57
  high fiber, 68
breakfast, plan for, 46–48
breast-feeding, 206, 213, 218–19
"brittle" diabetics, 128–29
bullosa diabeticorum, 187
Bursell, Sven-Erik, 171
Butazoladine, 195

calcitonin nasal spray, 182
calcium supplements, 70
California Institute of Technology, 141
calories, 32
  amount needed per day, 55
  defined, 35
capsaicin, 182
captopril (Capoten), 175
carbamazepine, 181
carbohydrates, 31–82
  in alcoholic drinks, 76, 77
  complex, 39–45
  defined, 34, 37
  effect on blood sugar, 36–40
  exercise and, 59
  list of 10-gram foods, 41–42
  list of 15-gram foods, 42–43
  simple, 38
  values of foods, listed, 80–82
cardiovascular disease, 13, 161–62
  cholesterol and, 55–56
Cardura, 179
carob, 73
cataracts, 172–73
catsup, 60
cereals, 46, 47–48
  with high sugar content, 60
cesarean delivery, 217
Charcot's foot, 181
cheese, 55, 56, 61
Chemstrip bG, 137–38
Chinese restaurants, 63, 238

chocolate, 22
cholesterol, 55–57, 159, 160, 162–63
chromium picolinate, 69–70
cigarette smoking, 74, 163, 167
cirrhosis of the liver, 20
Cisapride, 178
Clonidine, 182
cocaine, 75
cocoa, 22
codeine, 179
coffee, 22, 47
cold
  effect on insulin needs, 92
  insulin reactions and, 147–48
coma
  diabetic, 8, 10
  hyperosmolar neoketotic, 155, 178
  see also acidosis
Compazine, 192, 193
complications. See diabetic complications
conception, 207
constipation, 179
contraception, 224–25
coronary heart disease, death from, with high blood sugar levels, 30
cortisone, 117, 186
  insulin requirements and, 195
cost of diabetes, 4
cough medicines, 193
Coumadin, 195
Coxsackie B$_4$ virus, 11
cranberry juice, 60
creams, moisturizing, 187
cytoplasmic pancreatic-islet-cell antibodies, 12

decaffeinated beverages, 47
dehydration, 24
delta cells, 7
dental hygiene, 183–85
Desaryl, 177

dexamethasone, 195
dextrin, 37
dextrose, 73
DHEA, 71
Diabeta, 96, 98, 101
Diabetes Control and Complica-
    tions Trial (DCCT), 159
diabetes mellitus
    causes of, 11–12
    control of, 13–14
    control of, with exercise, 83–94
    defined, 5
    diagnosis of, 23–30
    diet for. See diet for diabetes and
        hypoglycemia
    genetic factors in, 9, 10, 11
    living with, 14–16
    preventing, 239–42
    research on, 109
    risk factors for, 12–14, 30, 240,
        241
    statistics, 3–5, 10, 14, 215–16
    symptoms of, 24
    three "T's," 157
Diabetes Prevention Program,
    240
diabetic complications, 4, 13,
    158–87
    acidosis, 153–57
    arteriosclerosis, 98
    cardiovascular, 161–62
    chances of acquiring, 161
    dermal, 185–87
    diabetic coma, 8, 10, 32
    drugs under investigation, 160
    exercise for prevention of, 83–84
    kidney problems, 174–76
    lowering the risk of, 14
    neuropathy, 176–82
    periodontal, 182–83
    podiatric, 177, 180, 197–98,
        236
    preventive measures, 83–84,
        159–60, 162–65

urinary, 179–80
visual, 165–74. See also
    retinopathy
diabetic research, 240–41
diabetics
    age at onset of, 9, 10
    brittle, 128–29
    gestational, 141, 208, 209–10,
        240
    pre-, defined, 210
    type 1, defined, 4, 10–11
    type 2, defined, 4, 8–10
diabetologist, 207, 208
Diabinese, 76, 78, 96, 98, 101
diagnosis of diabetes mellitus,
    23–30
diarrhea, 178, 179, 192–93, 236
diet for diabetes and hypoglycemia,
    19, 21–22, 31–82, 242
    artificial sweeteners in, 71–72
    calories in, 35, 55
    carbohydrates in, 36–37, see
        also carbohydrates
    "cheating" on, 65
    cholesterol in, 55–57
    complex carbohydrates in,
        39–45
    "dietetic" foods, 72–73
    equivalents, 45
    fast foods in, 57
    fasting, 64–65
    fiber in, 66–68
    food components in, 34–35
    foods to avoid in, 38–39
    free foods, 50–51
    fructose in, 73
    grams in, 35–36
    high-protein diets, 79
    hints for, 57–59
    in hospitals, 60
    importance of, 31–32
    insulin users, tips for, 40, 45–46,
        47, 49, 50, 53, 54, 62–63,
        64–65

low-potassium diets, 79
low-salt diets, 79
meal planning, 45–51
meat and fish, 54–55
oral agents and, 101–2
pitfalls in, 59–61
restaurant food in, 45, 63–64
rules for, 52
salad dressings, 62
snacks, 49–50
sugar in the diet, 39
timing of meals, 62–63
vegetarian, 78–79
vitamins and supplements in, 68–71
weight loss and, 51–54
"dietetic" foods, 37, 72–73
diets, rated, 78–79
Dilantin, 155, 177–78, 184, 195
dinner, plan for, 48–49
disaccharide, 73
diuretics, insulin sensitivity and, 242
dizziness, insulin reactions and, 147
double vision, 172, 178
drugs
    diabetes and, 12, 74–75, 155
    insulin reactions and, 147
    interactions with, 195–96
    interactions with oral agents, 105
    to prevent diabetic complications, 160
    for weight loss, 53
    without sugar, 193
"dry foot," 180
ducitol, 73
"dumping syndrome," 20
Dupuytren's contracture, 178
Dymelor, 96, 97, 101

eggs, 47
Elavil, 177

electrical spinal cord stimulation (ESCS), 182
emotions, insulin reactions and, 146–47
end-stage kidney disease, 13, 14
erythromycin, 179
estriol levels, 217
estrogen replacement therapy, 225–26
evening primrose oil, 182
exercise, 15, 83–94, 204
    aerobic, 90
    alcohol and, 93–94
    best time for, 89
    calorie usage table, 94
    company while exercising, 92
    complications prevented by, 83–84, 85, 164, 174
    contraindications to, 90–91
    diabetes controlled by, 85–86, 163, 241–42
    effect on NIDDM, 9
    effect on retinopathy, 85, 91
    frostbite dangers, 93
    hypoglycemia and, 22
    insulin injections and, 91
    insulin reactions and, 144, 145
    insulin users, tips for, 86–92
    snacks during, 88–89
    taking extra carbohydrates, 59
    testing blood beforehand, 89–90
    wardrobe for, 92
    weight loss and, 53–54
    while ill, 193
eyes. See vision, effects on by diabetes

fast foods, 57
fasting, 64–65
fasting blood-sugar levels, 7, 17–18, 28, 29, 132
fasting plasma glucose test, 26

fats
cholesterol and, 56–57
defined, 35
feet, diabetic's care of, 197–204
examination of the feet, 198–99,
200
exercise and, 204
footware, 201–2
important don'ts, 203–4
neuropathy and, 177, 180, 198
pedicures, 200–201
skin care, 200
types of problems, 197–98
washing, 199–200
fertility, effects of diabetes on, 223
fetal survival rate, in diabetic
mothers, 205
fiber in the diet, 35, 44, 66–68, 242
fish, 55
Flagyl, 179
floaters, 173–74
fluids, lost in exercising, replacing,
89
foods
to avoid, in foreign countries, 236
components of, 34–35
to eat while ill, 191–92
footware, 201–2
foreign countries, insulin in, 128
foreign languages, dietetic phrases
in, 231
free foods, 50–51
frostbite, 93
fructosamine test, 140–41
fructose, 37, 57, 73
"fruit drinks," 60
fruit juices, 46, 58, 60–61
fruits, 43, 58
high fiber, 68
fungal infections, 185, 193

GAD 65 antibodies, 240
gall bladder disease, 226
gastrointestinal tract, effect of
neuropathy on, 178–79

genetic factors, 9, 10, 11
genetic markers, 12
Gennid Study, 241
German measles, 11
gestational diabetes, 141, 208,
209–10, 240
ginseng, 75
glargine, 108, 116
glaucoma, 168, 170, 173
glimepiride, 101
glipizides, 98, 101
glitazones, 100
glucagon, 7
glucagon injection kit, 117
gluconeogenesis, 8, 75
Glucophage, 19, 96, 99–100, 101,
190, 241
glucose, 7, 25, 73, 84
concentrations, normal vs.
diabetic, 8
role of in the body, 5–6
glucose tolerance, impaired (IGT),
29, 30, 240–41
glucose tolerance test (GTT), 21,
25, 27
interpreting, 27–28
during pregnancy, 210
typical test results, 29
Glucotrol, 96, 98, 101
glyburides, 98, 101
"glycemic index," 39
glycogen, 5, 7, 37, 84
glycohemoglobin test (HbA1c),
26–27, 139–40
glycosaminoglycans, 175
glycosuria, 131–32
Glynase Prestab, 96, 98,
101
Glyset, 100, 101
grams, defined, 35–36
gum disease, 182–83

hamburgers, 57
Harold Rifkin Family Acquisition
Centers, 241

HbA1c: the glycohemoglobin test, 26–27, 139–40
HDL, 70, 75, 163–64, 242
    effects of exercise on, 83
    effects of oral agents on, 99
"health foods," 61
heart disease. *See* cardiovascular disease
heat
    effect on insulin needs, 92
    insulin reactions and, 147–48
heroin, 75
high blood pressure. *See* hypertension
high-protein diets, 79
Hispanic Americans, rates of diabetes among, 5
HLA genes, 12
hormone replacement therapy (HRT), 225–26
hormones, blood sugar regulated by, 7
hospitals, diets in, 60
Humalog (insulin lispro), 49, 110–11, 112
Humulin, 112
hunger, excessive, 24
hydramnios, 211
hyperglycemia, defined, 5
hyperlipidemia, 162
hyperosmolar neoketotic coma, 155
hypertension, 13, 162–63, 167, 175
hypoglycemia, 8, 17–22
    causes of, 19–20
    defined, 5, 17
    diagnosis of, 21
    diet for. *See* diet for diabetes and hypoglycemia
    glucose tolerance test results, 29
    oral agents and, 99
    symptoms, 18
"hypoglycemia unawareness," 147
hypoglycemic reactions. *See* insulin reactions

hypotension, orthostatic, 180
Hytrin, 179

ibuprofen, 176
ILA2 antibodies, 240
impaired glucose tolerance test (IGT), 29, 30, 240–41
impotence, 220–22
Inderal, 147, 195
infections
    of the feet, 198
    fungus and yeast, 185, 193, 223
inherited tendency to diabetes, 9, 10, 11
injections
    choosing the spot, 119–20, 146
    exercise and, 91
    filling the syringe, 118
    injecting the insulin, 120–21
    instructions for, 117–21
    materials needed for, 118
    mixed doses, 124
    mixing two insulins in one syringe, 118–19
    multiple, plan for, 124–25
    poor vision and, 121
    split doses, 124, 213
injuries, 194
"Instant Glucose," 149, 237
insulin, 4–5, 15, 107–29
    allergic reactions to, 116
    animal, 108, 116
    discovery of, 107–8
    double doses, 127
    effects of exercise on, 84
    emergencies, preparing for, 128
    fast-acting, 110–11
    in foreign countries, 128
    forgetting to take, 126–27
    frequency of blood tests and, 133
    function of, 7–8
    future types of, 109
    guide to, 112
    Humalog (insulin lispro), 110–11, 112

insulin *(cont'd)*
  human, 6–7, 108, 116
  injection instructions, 117–21
  intermediate-acting, 87, 111
  Lente, 111, 112
  long-acting, 111, 112
  manufacture of by the pancreas,
    6–7
  mixed doses, 124
  multiple injections, plan for,
    124–25
  NPH, 111, 112, 116, 146
  overproduction of, 19–20
  pen injectors, 115–16
  premixed, 112
  Regular, 87, 110, 111, 112, 116,
    189
  requirements while ill, 188,
    189–91, 193–94
  resistance to, 117
  skipping doses, 54
  solubility of, 108
  split doses, 124, 127, 213
  storage of, 121–22
  strengths of, 113
  during surgery, 194
  synthetic, 108
  syringes and needles, 114–15
  traveling with, 227, 229–30,
    236–38
  types of, 110–12
  Ultralente, 111, 112
insulin atrophy, 186–87
insulin hypertrophy, 186–87
insulin inhaler, 109
insulin pump, 122–24, 214, 225, 229
insulin reactions, 142–52
  acidosis *vs.,* 151–52
  causes of, 144, 146–48
  diabetic complications and, 164
  diet therapy or oral agents, 143
  exercise and, 86–87, 89
  nighttime, 148
  during pregnancy, 212
  prevention of, 144–46

  symptoms of, 143–44
  training other people what to
    do, 150–51
  treatment for, 148–50
  without warning, 150
insulin users
  diet tips for, 62–63
  exercise tips for, 86–92
  fasting and, 64–65
  ill, tips for, 188, 189–91, 193–94
  pregnant, 211–14
  travel tips for, 227, 229–30,
    232–38
insulin-dependent diabetes mellitus
    (IDDM). *See* type 1 diabetes
islet-cell antibodies, 240
islets of Langerhans, 7
Italian restaurants, 63–64
IUDs, 225

Japanese restaurants, 64, 238
jaundice, in the newborn, 215
Joslin Diabetes Center, 109, 168,
    171, 205
Juvenile Diabetes Foundation, 15,
    189, 208
"juvenile-onset" diabetes. *See* type
    1 diabetes

Keto-Diastix, 135–36
ketones. *See* acetone (ketones)
ketosis. *See* acidosis
kidney problems, 13, 14, 159,
    174–76
  during pregnancy, 211

labels on food, interpreting, 73–74
lactobacillus, 193
lactose, 73
Lamisil, 185
Lantus, 108, 112, 116
laser treatment, diabetic glaucoma,
    170
LDL, 163–64
  effect of exercise on, 83

effect of oral agents on, 99
legumes, 68
Lentard, 230
Lente, 112, 146
leptin, 53
lifestyle, and diabetes, 15–16, 241
lignin, 66
lipoprotein lipase, 57
liver, function of, 7
liver disease, 20
Lomotil, 179, 192
Lopressor, 147
lotions, moisturizing, 187
low-potassium diets, 79
low-salt diets, 79
lunches, plan for, 48–49
LY33531, 160, 175

magnesium, 70, 171
maltose, 37
mannitol, 37, 73
margarine, 56
marijuana, 74, 174
maturity-onset diabetes. *See* type 2
    diabetes
meal plans, for diet, 45–51
mean blood glucose (MBG), 26–27
meat, 54–55
MedicAlert, 152
medications. *See* drugs
Medrol, 195
meglinitides, 100
melatonin, 71
menstruation, insulin reactions
    and, 146
metformin, 96, 99–100, 101, 241
Mexiletene, 182
microalbuminurea (PKC-B), 160,
    176
microaneurysms, 166, 168
Micronase, 96, 98, 101
Middle Eastern restaurants, 64
Midodrine, 180
miglitol, 100, 101
milk, 40, 43, 61, 219

milk imitations, 60
minerals, importance of, 35
miscarriages, 211
mistakes in dosage, 127
monosaccharides, 37
Monotard, 230
morning sickness, 212
mumps, 11
myonisotol, 181

Nachtigall, Lila, 225
narcotics, diabetes and, 75
nateglinide, 100, 101
National Institutes of Health, 239
Native Americans, rates of diabetes
    among, 5, 11, 12, 14
nausea, 192
    during pregnancy, 212
necrobiosis lipoidica diabeticorum
    (NLD), 186
needles, 114–15
    disposal of, 126
nerve disease, 13, 14
nerve growth factor (NGF), 182
neuropathy, 159, 176–82, 223
    causes of, 176–77
    defined, 176
    effect of on the body, 177–78
    foot ulcers, 180
    numbness in legs and feet,
        177–78
    rare conditions caused by, 180–81
    symptoms, 176
    treatments, 181–82
Neurotonin, 177
newborns, of diabetic mothers,
    215–18
NLD, 186
nocturia, 24
nocturnal penile tumescence (NPT)
    assessment, 221
"noncaloric foods," 73
noninsulin-dependent diabetes
    mellitus (NIDDM). *See* type 2
    diabetes

nonsulfonylurea oral agents, 96, 99–100
Novolin, 112
Novolog, 112
NPH, 111, 112, 116, 146
Nurses' Health Study, 241
nuts, 58

obesity, 6, 9, 11, 162, 240
oligosaccharides, 37, 39–40
oral agents, 10, 86, 95–106
    blood tests while taking, 102–3
    contraindications to, 99–100
    death from heart disease and, 97
    diet and, 101–2
    drug interactions, 105, 195–96
    frequency of blood tests and, 133
    during illness, 103
    long-term effectiveness of, 105–6
    during pregnancy, 206, 219
    reactions to, 104–5, 143
    safety of, 96–97
    side effects of, 99–100, 104
    taking while ill, 190
    traveling with, 229, 230, 233, 238
    types of, 96–101
oranges, 36
Orinase, 96, 97, 101
orthostatic hypotension, 186
"ostrich syndrome," 160
oxytocin challenge test, 217–18

pain, neuropathic, 177, 181
pancreas
    function of, 6–7
    role of, in hypoglycemia, 20
pancreatic transplants, 109
pancreatitis, 12
Paris Prospective Study, 30
pasta, 45
pedicures, 200–201
pen injectors, 115–16, 229
penile implants, 222
periodontal disease, 182–85

photocoagulation, 169–70
pioglitazone, 100, 101
pizza, 57
polydipsia, 24
polyphagia, 24
polysaccharides, 37, 39–40
polyuria, 24
potassium, 79
Pramalintide, 19
Prandin, 100, 101
Precose, 19, 96, 100, 101, 190
prediabetics, defined, 210
predictors of diabetes, 12–14, 30, 240, 241
prednisone, 155, 195
pregnancy, 205–19
    blood-sugar control and, 206
    breast-feeding, 218–19
    choosing your obstetrician, 207–8
    classification of diabetic women, 208–9
    complications in, 210–11, 216–18
    conception, 207
    diet in, 214–15
    fetal survival rate, 205
    gestational diabetes, 208, 209–10
    insulin reactions in, 146
    insulin use in, 206, 209, 211–14
    oral agents and, 206, 219
    planning ahead, 206–7
    prediabetics and, 210
    saccharine as dangerous in, 72
    sugar in urine and, 25
    testing for maturity of fetus, 218
    tests during, 210
proliferative retinopathy, 168–69
Prolixin, 177
Propulsid, 178
prostaglandin E-1, 222
protease inhibitors, 155
protein
    defined, 34–35
    high-protein diets, 79
protein PC-1, 9

racial distribution of diabetes, 5
Rapitard, 230
Reglan, 178, 179
Regular insulin, 87, 110, 111, 112, 116, 189
renal thresholds, 131–32
repaglinide, 100, 101
research, diabetic, 240–41
respiratory distress syndrome (RDS), 218
restaurants, 63–64
    Chinese, 63, 238
    fast food, 57
    Italian, 63–64
    Japanese, 64, 238
    Middle Eastern, 64
retina, detached, 169
retinitis proliferans, 168–69
retinopathy, 14, 54, 85, 91, 159, 165–66
    aspirin use and, 165
    background retinopathy, defined, 166
    eye check-ups, importance of, 168–69
    preventive measures, 167, 170–71
    proliferative, 168–69
    treatment, 169–70
retrograde ejaculation, 223
Rezulin, 100, 241
risk factors for diabetes, 12–14, 30, 240, 241
Robitussin, 193
rosiglitazone, 100, 101

saccharin (Sweet'n Low, Sweet Magic, Sugar Twin, Sucaryl), 72
salad dressings, 62
salt, 79
sauces, 45
saunas, 147, 203
second-voided urine specimen, 134
selenium, 70

sex and the diabetic, 220–26
    contraception, 224–25
    effects on fertility, 223
    hormone replacement, 225–26
    impotence, 181, 220–22
    insulin needs, 225
    women, 223–24
sickness, 188–96
    acidosis and, 155
    diarrhea, 192–93
    drug interactions, 195–96
    easy-to-eat foods, 191–92
    injuries, 194
    insulin requirements, 188, 189–91, 193–94
    rules for, 189–94
    surgery and, 194–95
    urine/blood tests, 189–90
    vomiting, 192
sildenafil, 222
skin, diabetic's care of, 185–87, 200
smoking and diabetes, 74, 163, 167
snacks, 49–50
    emergency, 233, 234–35
    during exercise, 88–89
somatostatin, 7
sonography, 218
sorbitol, 37, 73
"sorbitol pathway," 176–77
soups, 43, 58–59
soy sauce, 50
spotted leg syndrome, 185–86
starch, 37
Starlix, 100
statistics, 3–5, 10, 14, 215–16
stress, 11, 13, 146, 162
strokes, 13, 162
sucrose, 37
Sudafed, 193
sugar
    forms of, 73
    hidden, 60–61, 73–74
    in medications, 193
    rapidly absorbed, 149

sugarless foods, 37
sulfonamides, 195
sulfonylurea oral agents, 96, 97–100
sunburn, 236
surfactant, 218
surgery, 194–95
sweating, abnormal, 180
sweeteners, artificial, 60, 71–72
syringes, 114–15, 230
    disposal of, 126
syrup, 47

tea, 22, 47
teeth and gums, diabetic's care of,
    183–85
Tegretol, 181
Tenormin, 147
test strips, 137–38
testosterone levels, 222
tetracycline, 179
thirst, as diabetic symptom, 24
Tigan, 192
Tolinase, 96, 97–98, 101
Tolrestat, 182
tomato sauce, 41, 45
tomatoes, 59
toxemia, 211
travel tips, 227–38
    after arriving, 235–36
    changing time zones, 232–35
    diabetic phrases in foreign
        languages, 231
    dining late, 237–38
    finding a doctor, 231–32
    insulin concerns, 227, 229–30,
        232–38
    keeping feet protected, 236
    list of suggestions, 228
    preparing for problems,
        228–29
    what not to eat or drink, 236
Triaminic, 193
triglycerides, 55, 56
    effect of oral agents on, 99
troglitazone, 100, 241

tumors, 12
    pancreatic, 20
twins, and risk factor for diabetes, 13
type 1 diabetes, 10–11
    glucose tolerance test results, 29
    preventing, 239–40
    risk of developing, 240
    statistical facts about, 4–5
type 2 diabetes, 4, 8–10
    glucose tolerance test results, 29
    insulin resistance, 100
    preventing, 240–41
    risk factors, 30, 241
    statistical facts about, 3–5
    symptoms, 9

ulcers
    neuropathic foot, 180, 204
    skin, 186
Ultralente, 112
Ultratard, 230
units of insulin, defined, 112–13
United Kingdom Prospective Dia-
    betes Study, 100
University Group Diabetes
    Program, 96
uremia, 175
urinary infections, 179–80, 211, 223
urination, excessive, 24
urine testing, 24–25, 131–32,
    134–35, 211

vaginal dryness, 224
vaginal infections, 185, 193, 223
vanadium, 71
vegetables, 43–44
    high fiber, 67
vegetarian diets, 78–79
Viagra, 222
viruses, as cause of type 1, 11–12,
    240
vision, effects on by diabetes,
    165–74, 178
    blurred vision, 171–72
    cataracts, 172–73

chances of developing eye problems, 165–66
double vision, 172, 178
effects of marijuana on vision, 174
floaters, 173–74
glaucoma, 173
retinopathy, 165–71, 174
vitamin $B_1$, 68–69, 181
vitamin $B_6$, 69
vitamin $B_{12}$, 181
vitamin C, 69, 170, 181
vitamin E, 69, 159, 168, 171, 175, 181
vitamins, nutritional need for, 35, 68–71
vitrectomy, 170
vomiting, 192, 238
  insulin reactions and, 147

wardrobe, for exercising, 92
water, importance of, 35
weight loss
  diet for, 51–54
  excessive, 24
wheat germ, 69
White, Priscilla, 208

xanthines, hypoglycemia due to, 22
xanthomatosis, eruptive, 187
xylitol, 73

yeast infections, 185
yogurt, 41–42, 193
yohimbine, 222

zinc, 70–71
Zostrex, 182

# ABOUT THE AUTHORS

STANLEY MIRSKY, M.D., F.A.C.P., Diplomate of Internal Medicine, is associate clinical professor of metabolic diseases at the Mount Sinai School of Medicine in New York, and is on the staffs of Mount Sinai and Lenox Hill Hospitals. A former president of the American Diabetes Association, New York Diabetes affiliate, he has been a member of the board of directors of the New York Diabetes Association.

Dr. Mirsky is also on the board of directors of the Joslin Diabetes Center, Inc., in Boston, and he is the chairman of the Nutrition Committee of Lenox Hill Hospital. A member of the Medical Advisory Board of the New York Chapter of the Juvenile Diabetes Foundation, he received the Humanitarian Award of the Juvenile Diabetes Foundation, New York Chapter, in 1994.

A Phi Beta Kappa graduate of the University of Michigan, he also graduated from Northwestern University Medical School and was a captain in the U.S. Air Force.

JOAN RATTNER HEILMAN is a respected journalist and author who has written more than a dozen books and hundreds of magazine and newspaper articles, many of them on health and medicine. A member of the American Society of Journalists and Authors and the Authors Guild, she is a graduate of Smith College and a former magazine editor. Collaborating with noted physicians, she has coauthored many books, including *Estrogen: The Facts Can Change Your Life*; *What Every Woman Should Know: Staying Healthy After 40*; *Having a Cesarean Baby*; *The Complete University Medical Diet*; *The Complete Book of Midwifery*; and *Growing Up Thin*.

## A B O U T   T H E   T Y P E

This book was set in Sabon, a typeface designed by the well-known German typographer Jan Tschichold (1902–74). Sabon's design is based upon the original letter forms of Claude Garamond and was created specifically to be used for three sources: foundry type for hand composition, Linotype, and Monotype. Tschichold named his typeface for the famous Frankfurt typefounder Jacques Sabon, who died in 1580.